A FEAST OF INFORMATION—
for people who love to eat but need to know
the sodium count of their meals.

**THE BARBARA KRAUS 1984 SODIUM
GUIDE TO BRAND NAMES & BASIC FOODS**
lists thousands of basic and ready-to-eat foods
from appetizers to desserts—carry it to the
supermarket, to the restaurant, to the beach, to
the coffee cart, and on trips. Flip through these
fact-filled pages and you'll be able to keep track
of your sodium intake as it adds up.

The Barbara Kraus
1984 Sodium
Guide to
Brand Names and
Basic Foods

SIGNET Books by Barbara Kraus

The Barbara Kraus 1984 Sodium Guide to Brand Names and Basic Foods

With *A Note on Sodium* by
Reva T. Frankle, Ed.D., R.D.
Director of Nutrition,
Weight Watchers International, Inc.

Ⓢ
A SIGNET BOOK
NEW AMERICAN LIBRARY

*For Danny Gorman and
Theresa Kelly*

Foreword

The composition of the foods we eat is not static: it changes from time to time. In the case of *brand-name* products, manufacturers alter their recipes to reflect the availability of ingredients, advances in technology, or improvements in formulae. Each year new products appear on the market and some old ones are discontinued.

On the other hand, information on *basic foods* such as meats, vegetables, and fruits may also change as a result of the development of better analytical methods, different growing conditions, or new marketing practices. These changes, however, are usually relatively small as compared with those in manufactured products.

Some differences may be found between the values in this book and those appearing on the product labels. This is usually due to the fact that the Food and Drug Administration permits manufacturers to round the figures reported on labels. The data in this book are reported as calculated without rounding. If large differences between the two sets of values are noted, they may be due to changes in product formulae, and in those cases the label data should be used.

For all these reasons, a book of nutritive values of foods must be kept up to date by a periodic reviewing and revision of the data presented.

Therefore, this handy sodium counter will provide each year the most current and accurate estimates available.

Good eating in 1984! For 1985, we'll pick up the new products, drop any has-beens, and make whatever other changes are necessary.

Barbara Kraus

A Note on Sodium

by Reva T. Frankle, Ed.D., R.D.
Director of Nutrition,
Weight Watchers International, Inc.

"Excess of salty flavor hardens the pulse."
*The Yellow Emperor's Classic
of Internal Medicine,* circa 1000 B.C.

Salt has always been considered the king of seasoning. Historically, it has been associated with social status and wealth. In previous centuries, the most important guests at the table were seated "above the salt," and salt provided the root for the word "salary" (literally, money earned for the purchase of salt).

Today, however, salt's age-old preeminence is being challenged. Research has linked excessive salt consumption with hypertension (high blood pressure), an important risk factor in cardiovascular disease. For this reason, the government's "Dietary Guidelines for Americans," published by the Department of Agriculture in 1980, recommends avoiding too much sodium.

It has been estimated that Americans consume about 10 to 12 grams of salt daily, which amounts to about 2 to 2½ teaspoons. Since salt (sodium chloride) is about 40 percent sodium, this level of salt intake is equal to between 4 and 4½ grams of sodium per day. Where does this salt come from? Of the 10 to 12 grams of salt consumed daily, approximately one-third occurs naturally in foods, one-third comes from salt-containing ingredients added to foods during processing, and one-third represents discretionary salt added by the consumer (from the salt shaker during cooking and at the table). Drinking water also contains sodium, the amount varying from locale to locale.

Though there has been much discussion recently about the dangers of salt, let's not lose sight of the fact that sodium, a naturally occurring constituent of all foods, is an essential nutrient. Sodium is a key element in the regulation of body water and plays a vital role in the acid-base balance of the body. In fact sodium, like chloride, is indispensable for many body processes, including the conduction of nerve impulses, heart action, and the function of certain enzyme systems. It's the *excessive* intake of salt that is being questioned.

Today, about 20 percent of the American population has high blood pressure—a primary cause of the 500,000 cases of stroke and the 1.2 million heart attacks that occur each year. High blood pressure is painless, "silent," and therefore often ignored until a complicating event causes it to manifest itself. Yet with proper diet and medical treatment, high blood pressure can be controlled and its complications prevented. For many Americans who suffer this silent disease, a reduced sodium intake is critical. In addition, those people who tend to retain body fluids due to kidney, heart, and liver conditions may want to check with their physicians about a decreased sodium intake. Available evidence indicates that restricting sodium to approximately 3.5 grams of salt per day will effect a slight reduction in blood pressure among moderately hypertensive adults. Several very carefully controlled studies of severely hypertensive adults have shown that sodium must be restricted to 200 milligrams (0.5 grams of salt) per day in order to achieve a significant reduction in blood pressure.

Although efforts to correlate salt intake with the incidence of hypertension have not provided definitive evidence of a causal relationship, nonetheless, evidence seems to indicate there is no risk in lowering present intakes of dietary sodium. The possible link between sodium intake and hypertension has become an issue of increasing concern in the United States. Since hypertension is a potent risk factor for coronary heart disease and stroke, its control is a major health concern. Current treatment of hypertension requires a change in lifestyle—particularly in terms of dietary habits.

A discussion of dietary sodium is complicated. As you will learn as you use this book, some high-sodium foods do not taste salty or are not thought of as salty. For example, an analysis of a serving of fast-food french fries shows 115 milligrams of sodium per serving, whereas a serving of cherry pie has nearly four times this amount, or 450 milligrams.

As a public health nutritionist and a clinical dietitian, may I suggest that in place of salt you sometimes try seasoning foods with some of the following condiments and spices. Onion, garlic, lemon, lime, and vinegar are particularly useful, as are herbs and spices like allspice, aniseed, basil, bay leaf, caraway seed, cardamon, cayenne pepper, celery seed, chili powder, cinnamon, cloves, curry powder, dill seed, fennel seed, garlic, ginger, mace, marjoram, mint, mustard (dry), mustard seed, nutmeg, onion powder, oregano, parsley, pepper, poppy seed, poultry seasoning, rosemary, saffron, sage, sesame seed, tarragon, thyme, turmeric, and vanilla.

Agreed, the sodium intake of Americans is excessive. Since there is no reason to believe that reducing sodium chloride intake would be harmful for healthy persons, and it may even help prevent hypertension in some people, it is time to evaluate our sodium intake. The consumer can meet the challenge of decreasing sodium intake by being aware of the sodium content of foods and using discretion with the salt shaker. There is no specific recommended amount or safety level, but the National Research Council suggests that the estimated safe and adequate daily dietary intake of sodium is about 1100 to 3000 milligrams (1.1 to 3.3 grams). Limiting salt intake to

3 grams per day would allow for some salt to be used in cooking but none at the table.

Industry is responding. Sodium-containing substances such as salt are added to foods for three basic reasons: 1) to provide and enhance flavors in foods, 2) to develop and maintain expected characteristics of foods such as texture and freshness, and 3) as a preservative. Gradual reduction, appropriate for some foods, is taking place. Industry is experimenting with safe new processes for the use of salt, with reduced sodium formulas, and with the use of alternatives to sodium-containing ingredients. Gradual reduction will allow time for industry to determine the microbiologic safety of certain reduced-sodium products.

FDA is working with the processed-food industry on a voluntary basis to lower the sodium content of foods they produce. (Sodium is used almost universally in the preserving and processing of food.) The Department of Health and Human Services is working to give consumers more information about the sodium content of foods they buy, and has said it "would like to see more public awareness in general about sodium and health."

Dietary change is the cornerstone of safe, effective, long-term blood pressure control. How fortunate that we now have *The Barbara Kraus Sodium Guide to Brand Names and Basic Foods,* a comprehensive and easy-to-use book that enables readers to estimate their daily salt intake and to plan a diet that is lower in sodium.

ABBREVIATIONS AND SYMBOLS

* = prepared as package directs[1]
< = less than
& = and
" = inch
canned = bottles or jars as well as cans
dia. = diameter
fl. = fluid
liq. = liquid
lb. = pound
med. = medium

oz. = ounce
pkg. = package
pt. = pint
qt. = quart
sq. = square
T. = tablespoon
Tr. = trace
tsp. = teaspoon
wt. = weight

Italics or name in parentheses = registered trademark, ®. All data not identified by company or trademark are based on material obtained from the United States Department of Agriculture or Health, Education and Welfare/Food and Agriculture Organization.

EQUIVALENTS

By Weight	*By Volume*
1 pound = 16 ounces	1 quart = 4 cups
1 ounce = 28.35 grams	1 cup = 8 fluid ounces
3.52 ounces = 100 grams	1 cup = ½ pint
	1 cup = 16 tablespoons
	2 tablespoons = 1 fluid ounce
	1 tablespoon = 3 teaspoons
	1 pound butter = 4 sticks or 2 cups

[1]If the package directions call for whole or skim milk, the data given here are for whole milk unless otherwise stated.

Food and Description	Measure or Quantity	Sodium (mgs.)

A

Food and Description	Measure or Quantity	Sodium (mgs.)
AC'CENT	¼ tsp.	129
ACEROLA, fresh, fruit	4 oz.	9
ALBACORE, raw, meat only	4 oz.	45
ALLSPICE (French's)	1 tsp.	1
ALMOND:		
Shelled, raw, natural with skins	1 oz.	1
Roasted, dry (Planters)	1 oz.	222
Roasted, oil (Fisher)	1 oz.	56
ALPHA-BITS, cereal (Post)	1 cup (1 oz.)	219
APPLE:		
Eaten with skin	2½" dia.	<1
Eaten without skin	2½" dia.	<1
Canned (Comstock):		
Rings, drained	1 ring	8
Sliced	⅙ of 21-oz. can	30
Dried (Del Monte)	1 cup	57
Frozen, sweetened	10-oz. pkg.	40
APPLE BROWN BETTY	1 cup	352
APPLE BUTTER (Smucker's) cider	1 T.	1
APPLE CIDER:		
Canned (Mott's) sweet	½ cup	1
*Mix, *Country Time*	8 fl. oz.	94
APPLE-CRANBERRY DRINK (Hi-C):		
Canned	6 fl. oz.	23
*Mix	6 fl. oz.	11
APPLE DRINK:		
Canned:		
Capri Sun, natural	6¾ fl. oz.	2
(Hi-C)	6 fl. oz.	12
*Mix (Hi-C)	6 fl. oz.	20
APPLE DUMPLINGS, frozen (Pepperidge Farm)	1 dumpling	235
APPLE, ESCALLOPED, frozen (Stouffer's)	4 oz.	50

Food and Description	Measure or Quantity	Sodium (mgs.)
APPLE-GRAPE JUICE, canned		
(Red Cheek)	6 fl. oz.	2
APPLE JACKS, cereal (Kellogg's)	1 cup (1 oz.)	125
APPLE JELLY:		
Sweetened (Smucker's)	1 T.	3
Dietetic (See APPLE SPREAD)		
APPLE JUICE:		
Canned:		
(Minute Maid)	6 fl. oz.	2
(Mott's)	6 fl. oz.	<10
(Red Cheek)	6 fl. oz.	2
Chilled (Minute Maid)	6 fl. oz.	2
*Frozen:		
(Minute Maid)	6 fl. oz.	2
(Seneca Foods) natural style,		
Vitamin C added	6 fl. oz.	1
APPLE PIE (See PIE, Apple)		
APPLE SAUCE:		
Regular:		
(Del Monte)	½ cup	1
(Mott's):		
Natural	½ cup	<5
With ground cranberries	½ cup	<5
(Stokely-Van Camp)	½ cup	32
Dietetic:		
(Diet Delight)	½ cup	5
(Featherweight) water pack	½ cup	<10
APPLE SPREAD, low sugar:		
(Diet Delight)	1 T.	25
(Featherweight):		
Regular	1 T.	40
Artificially sweetened	1 T.	41
(Slenderella)	1 T.	20
APPLE STRUDEL, frozen		
(Pepperidge Farm)	3-oz. serving	215
APRICOT:		
Fresh, whole	1 apricot	<1
Canned, regular pack:		
(Del Monte) whole, peeled	1 cup	36
(Libby's) halves, heavy syrup	1 cup	14
(Stokely-Van Camp)	1 cup	45
Canned, dietetic:		
(Del Monte) *Lite*	½ cup	2
(Diet Delight) syrup pack or water pack	½ cup	5

Food and Description	Measure or Quantity	Sodium (mgs.)
(Featherweight) juice pack or water pack	½ cup	< 10
(Libby's) Lite	½ cup	10
Dried:		
(Del Monte)	2-oz. serving	3
(Sun-Maid; Sunsweet)	¼ cup (1.7 oz.)	13
APRICOT LIQUEUR (DeKuyper)	1 fl. oz.	
APRICOT NECTAR:		
(Del Monte)	6 fl. oz.	8
(Libby's)	6 fl. oz.	5
APRICOT & PINEAPPLE PRESERVE OR JAM:		
Sweetened (Smucker's)	1 T.	3
Dietetic (See APRICOT & PINEAPPLE SPREAD)		
APRICOT & PINEAPPLE SPREAD, low sugar:		
(Diet Delight)	1 T.	45
(Featherweight) artificially sweetened	1 T.	40–50
APRICOT SOUR COCKTAIL (National Distillers-*Duet*) 12½% alcohol	2 fl. oz.	TR.
ARBY'S:		
Beef & Cheese Sandwich	6 oz.	1220
Club Sandwich	9 oz.	1610
Ham'n Cheese	5½ oz.	1350
Roast Beef:		
Regular	5 oz.	880
Junior	3 oz.	530
Super	9¾ oz.	1420
Turkey Deluxe	8½ oz.	1220
ARTICHOKE:		
Boiled	15-oz. artichoke	128
Canned (Cara Mia) marinated, drained	6-oz. jar	94
Frozen (Birds Eye) deluxe, hearts	⅓ pkg.	40
ASPARAGUS:		
Boiled	1 spear (½″ dia. at base)	<1
Canned, regular pack, spears, solids & liq.:		
(Del Monte) green or white	1 cup	778
(Green Giant) green	8-oz. can	706
(Stokely-Van Camp)	1 cup	896
Canned, dietetic, solids & liq.:		
(Diet Delight)	½ cup	5

Food and Description	Measure or Quantity	Sodium (mgs.)
(Featherweight) cut spears	1 cup	<20
(S&W) *Nutradiet*	1 cup	<20
Frozen:		
(Birds Eye):		
Cuts	⅓ pkg.	<1
Spears, regular or jumbo deluxe	⅓ pkg.	4
(Green Giant) cuts, butter sauce	3 oz.	545
(McKenzie)	⅓ pkg.	4
ASPARAGUS SOUFFLE, frozen (Stouffer's)	4 oz.	440
AUNT JEMIMA SYRUP (See SYRUP)		
AVOCADO, all varieties	1 fruit	10
***AWAKE** (Birds Eye)	6 fl. oz.	15
AYDS:		
Butterscotch	1 piece	9
Vanilla	1 piece	12

B

BACON, broiled (Oscar Mayer):		
Regular slice	6-gram slice	114
Thick slice	1 slice	209
BACON BITS:		
(Betty Crocker) *Bac*Os*	1 tsp.	76
(Durkee) imitation	1 tsp.	229
(French's) imitation	1 tsp.	55
(Oscar Mayer) real	1 tsp.	54
BACON, CANADIAN, unheated:		
(Oscar Mayer) 93% fat free	.7-oz. slice	295
(Oscar Mayer) 93% fat free	1-oz. slice	393
BACON, SIMULATED, cooked:		
(Oscar Mayer) *Lean 'N Tasty*:		
Beef	1 slice	202
Pork	1 slice	220
(Swift) *Sizzlean*	1 strip	159
BAGEL:		
Egg	3-inch diameter, 1.9 oz.	245

Food and Description	Measure or Quantity	Sodium (mgs.)
Water	3-inch diameter, 1.9 oz.	205
BAKING POWDER: (Featherweight) low sodium, cereal free	1 tsp.	2
BAMBOO SHOOTS, canned, drained (La Choy)	½ cup	6
BANANA, medium	6.3-oz. banana (weighed unpeeled)	1
BANANA PIE (See PIE, Banana)		
BARBECUE SEASONING (French's)	1 tsp.	70
BARLEY, pearled (Quaker Scotch)	¼ cup	5
BASIL (French's)	1 tsp.	<1
BAY LEAF (French's)	1 tsp.	<1
B.B.Q. SAUCE & BEEF, frozen (Banquet) *Cookin' Bag*, sliced	5-oz. cooking bag	885
BEAN, BAKED:		
(USDA):		
With pork & molasses sauce	1 cup	969
With pork & tomato sauce	1 cup	1181
Canned:		
(B&M):		
Pea bean with pork in brown sugar sauce	8 oz.	848
Red kidney bean in brown sugar sauce	8 oz.	776
(Campbell):		
Home style	8-oz. can	1200
With pork & tomato sauce	8-oz. can	1100
(Libby's):		
Deep Brown, with pork & molasses sauce	½ of 14-oz. can	467
Deep Brown, vegetarian in tomato sauce	½ of 14-oz. can	714
(Van Camp) with pork	8 oz.	1005
BEAN, BARBECUE (Campbell)	7⅞-oz. can	1150
BEAN, BLACK, DRY	1 cup	56
BEAN, BROWN, DRY	1 cup	56
BEAN & FRANKFURTER, canned (Campbell) in tomato and molasses sauce	8-oz. can	1200
BEAN & FRANKFURTER DINNER, frozen:		
(Banquet)	10¾-oz. dinner	1995
(Morton)	10¾-oz. dinner	886
(Swanson) *TV Brand*	11¼-oz. dinner	1100

Food and Description	Measure or Quantity	Sodium (mgs.)
BEAN, GARBANZO, canned, dietetic (S&W) *Nutradiet*, low sodium	½ cup	<10
BEAN, GREEN:		
Boiled, 1½" to 2" pieces, drained	½ cup	4
Canned, regular pack:		
(Comstock) solids & liq.	½ cup	350
(Del Monte) French, drained	½ cup	461
(Green Giant) French or whole, solids & liq.	½ of 8½-oz. can	359
(Libby's) cut, solids & liq.	½ cup	333
(Libby's) French, solids & liq.	½ cup	335
(Stokely-Van Camp) solids & liq.	½ cup	103
(Sunshine) solids & liq.	½ cup	312
Canned, dietetic:		
(Diet Delight) solids & liq.	½ cup	5
(Featherweight) cut or French, solids & liq.	½ cup	<10
(S&W) *Nutradiet*, cut, solids & liq., low sodium	½ cup	<10
Frozen:		
(Birds Eye):		
Cut	⅓ pkg.	3
French, with mushrooms	⅓ pkg.	188
Italian style	⅓ pkg.	3
Whole, deluxe	⅓ pkg.	1
(Green Giant):		
With butter sauce	⅓ pkg.	297
With mushroom in cream sauce	⅓ pkg.	235
(McKenzie) cut or French style	⅓ pkg.	3
(Southland) cut or French style	⅕ of 16-oz. pkg.	3
BEAN, GREEN & MUSHROOM CASSEROLE, frozen (Stouffer's)	4¾ oz.	675
BEAN, GREEN WITH POTATOES, canned (Sunshine) solids & liq.	½ cup	398
BEAN, GREEN, PUREE, canned, dietetic (Featherweight)	1 cup	<10
BEAN, ITALIAN, canned (Del Monte) drained	½ cup	472
BEAN, KIDNEY:		
Canned, regular pack (Van Camp):		
Light	8 oz.	680
New Orleans style	8 oz.	793
Red	8 oz.	930
Canned, dietetic (S&W) *Nutradiet*, low sodium, solids & liq.	½ cup	<10

6

Food and Description	Measure or Quantity	Sodium (mgs.)
BEAN, LIMA:		
Boiled, without salt, drained	½ cup	<1
Canned, regular pack:		
(Del Monte) drained	½ cup	313
(Libby's) solids & liq.	½ cup	247
Canned, dietetic (Featherweight) solids & liq.	½ cup	25
Frozen:		
(Birds Eye) tiny, deluxe	⅓ pkg.	142
(Green Giant):		
In butter sauce	3 oz.	337
Harvest Fresh	4 oz.	345
(McKenzie):		
Baby Lima	⅓ pkg.	125
Fordhook	⅓ pkg.	71
Tiny	⅓ pkg.	144
(Southland) speckled butter	⅕ of 16-oz. pkg.	19
BEAN, PINTO (Del Monte) spicy	½ cup	497
BEAN, REFRIED, canned (Del Monte) regular	½ cup	459
BEAN, SALAD, canned (Green Giant)	4½-oz. serving	406
BEAN SOUP (See SOUP, Bean)		
BEAN SPROUT:		
Mung, raw	½ lb.	12
Mung, boiled, drained	¼ lb.	5
Canned (La Choy) drained	⅔ cup	27
BEAN, YELLOW OR WAX:		
Boiled, 1″ pieces, drained	½ cup	2
Canned, regular pack:		
(Comstock) solids & liq.	½ cup	350
(Del Monte) cut, solids & liq.	½ cup	331
(Festal) cut or French style, solids & liq.	½ cup	388
(Libby's) cut, solids & liq.	4 oz.	336
(Stokely-Van Camp) solids & liq.	½ cup	415
Canned, dietetic (Featherweight, cut, solids & liq.)	½ cup	<10
Frozen (McKenzie) cut	⅓ pkg.	1
BEEF, choice grade, medium done:		
Brisket, braised:		
Lean & fat	3 oz.	37
Lean only	3 oz.	51
Chuck, pot roast, lean only	3 oz.	51
Filet Mignon. See Steak, sirloin, lean		
Flank, braised, 100% lean	3 oz.	51

Food and Description	Measure or Quantity	Sodium (mgs.)
Ground:		
Regular, raw	½ cup	73
Regular, broiled	3 oz.	39
Lean, broiled	3 oz.	40
Rib, Roasted, lean & fat	3 oz.	51
Round:		
Broiled, lean & fat	3 oz.	51
Lean only	3 oz.	51
Steak, club, broiled:		
One 8-oz. steak (weighed without bone before cooking) will give you:		
Lean & fat	5.9 oz.	68
Lean only	3.4 oz.	68
Steak, porterhouse, broiled:		
One 16-oz. steak (Weighed with bone before cooking) will give you:		
Lean & fat	4 oz.	68
Lean only	5.9 oz.	72
BEEFAMATO COCKTAIL (Mott's)	6 fl. oz.	240
BEEF BOUILLON:		
(Herb-Ox):		
Cube	1 cube	500
Packet	1 packet	1040
MBT	1 packet	755
Low sodium (Featherweight)	1 tsp.	10
BEEF, CHIPPED:		
Frozen:		
(Banquet) creamed, *Cookin' Bag*	5-oz. pkg.	949
(Stouffer's) creamed	5½ oz.	900
(Swanson) creamed	10½ oz. entree	1545
BEEF DINNER or ENTREE, frozen:		
(Banquet):		
Regular	11-oz. dinner	1925
Chopped	11-oz. dinner	1934
Man Pleaser, sliced	20-oz. dinner	1371
(Morton):		
Regular	10-oz. dinner	824
Country Table sliced	14-oz. dinner	1313
(Swanson):		
Hungry Man, chopped	18-oz. dinner	1955
Hungry Man, sliced	12¼-oz. dinner	1345
TV Brand, chopped sirloin	10-oz. dinner	940
3-course	15-oz. dinner	1520

8

Food and Description	Measure or Quantity	Sodium (mgs.)
(Weight Watchers):		
Beefsteak, 2-compartment meal	9¾-oz. pkg.	961
Sirloin in mushroom sauce, 3-compartment meal	13-oz. pkg.	1609
BEEF, DRIED, canned (Swift)	¾-oz. serving	505
BEEF, GROUND, SEASONING MIX:		
*(Durkee):		
Regular	1 cup	799
With onion	1 cup	1099
(French's) with onion	1⅛-oz. pkg.	1760
BEEF HASH, ROAST, *Mary Kitchen*	7½-oz.	1327
BEEF PEPPER ORIENTAL, *canned (La Choy):*		
Regular	¾ cup	1285
Bi-pack	¾ cup	1095
BEEF PIE, frozen:		
(Banquet):		
Regular	8-oz. pie	908
Supreme	8-oz. pie	1245
(Morton)	8-oz. pie	1000
(Stouffer's)	10-oz. pie	1600
(Swanson):		
Regular	8-oz. pie	810
Hungry-Man	16-oz. pie	1490
BEEF SOUP (See SOUP, Beef)		
BEEF SPREAD, ROAST, CANNED (Underwood)	½ of 4¾-oz. can	515
BEEF STEW:		
Home recipe, made with lean beef chuck	1 cup	91
Canned, regular pack:		
Dinty Moore	7½-oz. serving	833
(Morton House)	⅓ of 24-oz. can	1114
(Swanson)	7⅝-oz. serving	890
Canned, dietetic (Featherweight)	7½ oz.	96
Frozen:		
(Banquet) *Buffet Supper*	2-lb. pkg.	5281
(Green Giant):		
Boil 'N Bag	9-oz. entree	274
Twin pouch, with noodles	9-oz. entree	637
(Stouffer's)	10 oz.	1675
BEEF STEW SEASONING MIX:		
*(Durkee)	1 cup	975
(French's)	1 pkg.	4590

9

Food and Description	Measure or Quantity	Sodium (mgs.)
BEEF STOCK BASE (French's)	1 tsp.	500
BEEF STROGANOFF, frozen (Stouffer's)	9¾ oz.	1300
***BEEF STROGANOFF SEASONING MIX** (Durkee)	1 cup	870
BEER & ALE:		
Regular:		
Black Horse Ale	8 fl. oz.	33
Budweiser	8 fl. oz.	12
Busch Bavarian	8 fl. oz.	12
Michelob	8 fl. oz.	12
Red Cap	8 fl. oz.	38
Light or low carbohydrate:		
Gablinger's	8 fl. oz.	14
Michelob, light	8 fl. oz.	12
Natural Light	8 fl. oz.	12
BEER, NEAR (Metbrew)	8 fl. oz.	18
BEET:		
Boiled, whole	2″ dia. beet	21
Boiled, sliced	½ cup	37
Canned:		
(Del Monte):		
Pickled, solids & liq.	½ cup	326
Sliced, drained	½ cup	316
(Greenwood):		
Harvard, solids & liq.	½ cup	350
Pickled, solids & liq.	½ cup	250
Pickled, with onion, solids & liq.	½ cup	250
(Libby's) Harvard, solids & liq.	½ cup	161
(Stokely-Van Camp) pickled, solids & liq.	½ cup	290
(Comstock) solids & liq.	½ cup	100
(Featherweight) sliced, solids & liq.	½ cup	55
(S&W) *Nutradiet*, sliced, solids & liq.	½ cup	40
BEET PUREE, canned, dietetic (Featherweight)	1 cup	120
***BIG H**, burger sauce (Hellmann's)	1 T.	143
***BIG MAC** (see *MC DONALD'S*)		
***BIG WHEEL** (Hostess)	1 cake	96
BLACKBERRY JELLY:		
Sweetened (Smucker's)	1 T.	4
Dietetic (See BLACKBERRY SPREAD)		

Food and Description	Measure or Quantity	Sodium (mgs.)
BLACKBERRY PRESERVE OR JAM:		
Sweetened (Smucker's)	1 T.	2
Dietetic:		
(Diet-Delight)	1 T.	19
(Featherweight)	1 T.	40
BLACKBERRY SPREAD, low sugar:		
(Diet Delight)	1 T.	45
(Featherweight)	1 T.	40
(Slenderella)	1 T.	16
BLACK-EYED PEAS:		
Canned (Sunshine) with pork, solids & liq.	½ cup	464
Frozen:		
(McKenzie)	⅓ pkg.	6
(Southland)	⅕ of 16-oz. pkg.	7
BLINTZE, frozen (King Kold) cheese	2½ oz. piece	250
BLOODY MARY MIX, dry (Bar-Tender's)	1 serving	510
BLUEBERRY, fresh, whole	½ lb.	2
BLUEBERRY PIE (See PIE, Blueberry)		
BLUEBERRY PRESERVE OR JAM, sweetened (Smucker's)	1 T.	6
BLUEFISH, broiled	3½″ × 3″ × ½″ piece	130
BODY BUDDIES, cereal (General Mills):		
Brown sugar & honey	1 cup	290
Natural fruit flavor	¾ cup	285
BOLOGNA:		
(Best's Kosher) Chub or sliced	1-oz. serving	443
(Hormel):		
Coarse ground, ring	1-oz. serving	320
Fine ground, ring	1-oz. serving	331
Meat	1-oz. slice	318
(Oscar Mayer):		
Beef	.8-oz. slice	239
Beef	1-oz. slice	295
Beef	1.3-oz. slice	394
Meat	.8-oz. slice	241
Meat	1-oz. slice	298
(Oscherwitz) chub or sliced	1-oz. serving	443
(Swift)	1-oz. slice	307
BOLOGNA & CHEESE (Oscar Mayer)	.8-oz. slice	244

Food and Description	Measure or Quantity	Sodium (mgs.)
BOO*BERRY, cereal (General Mills)	1 cup	210
BORSCHT, canned:		
Regular (Mother's) old fashioned	8-oz. serving	907
Dietetic or low calorie (Mother's):		
Artificially sweetened	8-oz. serving	943
Unsalted	8-oz. serving	51
BOSCO (See SYRUP)		
*BOWL O' NOODLES (Nestlé):		
Beef	1½-oz. envelope	950
Chicken	1½-oz. envelope	810
BOYSENBERRY JELLY, sweetened		
(Smucker's)	1 T.	3
BRAN, crude	1 oz.	3
BRAN, Miller's	1 oz.	6
BRAN BREAKFAST CEREAL:		
(Kellogg's):		
All Bran	⅓ cup	320
Bran Buds	⅓ cup	175
Cracklin' Bran	½ cup	170
40% bran flakes	¾ cup	220
Raisin	¾ cup	205
(Post) 40% bran flakes	⅔ cup	260
(Quaker) *Corn Bran*	⅔ cup	245
(Ralston-Purina):		
Bran Chex	⅔ cup	267
40% bran	¾ cup	294
Honey	⅞ cup	157
Raisin	¾ cup	286
BRAUNSCHWEIGER:		
(Oscar Mayer) chub	1 oz.	335
(Swift) 8-oz. chub	1 oz.	282
BRAZIL NUT, roasted (Fisher) salted	1-oz. serving	57
BREAD:		
Apple (Pepperidge Farm)	.9-oz. slice	105
Cinnamon (Pepperidge Farm)	.9-oz. slice	98
Corn & Molasses (Pepperidge Farm)	.9-oz. slice	130
Cracked wheat (Pepperidge Farm)	1 slice	130
Crispbread, *Wasa:*		
Mora	3.2-oz. slice	514
Rye, golden	.4-oz. slice	43
Rye, lite	.3-oz. slice	20
Sesame	.5-oz. slice	35
Sport	.4-oz. slice	66
Date Walnut (Pepperidge Farm)	.9-oz. slice	108
Flatbread, *Ideal:*		
Bran	.2-oz. slice	47

Food and Description	Measure or Quantity	Sodium (mgs.)
Extra thin	.1-oz. slice	25
Whole grain	.2-oz. slice	47
French:		
(Pepperidge Farm)	2-oz. slice	430
(Wonder)	1-oz. slice	170
Hillbilly	1-oz. slice	170
Hollywood, dark	1-oz. slice	162
Honey bran (Pepperidge Farm)	1.1-oz. slice	207
Honey, wheat berry (Arnold)	1.2-oz. slice	205
Italian (Pepperidge Farm)	2-oz. slice	320
Low sodium (Wonder)	1-oz. slice	3
Naturél (Arnold)	.9-oz. slice	43
Oatmeal (Pepperidge Farm)	1 slice	185
Orange & Raisin (Pepperidge Farm)	.9-oz. slice	88
Protogen Protein (Thomas')	.7-oz. slice	94
Pumpernickel:		
(Arnold)	1-oz. slice	230
(Levy's)	1.1-oz. slice	192
(Pepperidge Farm):		
Regular	slice	305
Party	slice	55
Raisin:		
(Arnold) tea	.9-oz. slice	112
(Pepperidge Farm)	.9-oz. slice	107
(Thomas')	.8-oz. slice	92
Roman Meal	1-oz. slice	159
Rye:		
(Arnold) Jewish	1.1-oz. slice	202
(Levy's) real	1.1-oz. slice	185
(Pepperidge Farm) family	1.1-oz. slice	242
(Wonder)	1-oz. slice	170
Sahara (Thomas'):		
Wheat	1-oz. piece	188
White	1-oz. piece	145
Sour dough, *Di Carlo*	1-oz. slice	156
Sprouted wheat (Pepperidge Farm)	.9-oz. slice	113
Vienna (Pepperidge Farm)	.9-oz. slice	175
Wheat:		
Fresh Horizons	1-oz. slice	148
Fresh & Natural	1-oz. slice	135
Home Pride	1-oz. slice	156
(Pepperidge Farm) family	1 slice	142
(Wonder) family	1-oz. slice	148
Wheatberry, *Home Pride*	1-oz. slice	163
Wheat Germ (Pepperidge Farm)	1 slice	145

13

Food and Description	Measure or Quantity	Sodium (mgs.)
White:		
(Arnold) *Brick Oven*	.8-oz. slice	102
Home Pride	1-oz. slice	149
(Pepperidge Farm):		
Large loaf	.9-oz. slice	175
Sandwich	.8-oz. slice	140
Sliced, 1-lb. loaf	.9-oz. slice	168
Toasting	1.2-oz. slice	240
(Wonder) regular	1-oz. slice	153
Whole wheat:		
(Arnold) *Brick Oven*	.8-oz. slice	210
(Arnold) *Measure Up*	.5-oz. slice	70
(Pepperidge Farm) thin slice	1 slice	145
(Thomas') 100%	.8-oz. slice	118
BREAD, CANNED, brown, plain or raisin (B&M)	½" slice	220
BREAD CRUMBS (Contadina) seasoned	½ cup	1580
***BREAD DOUGH**, frozen:		
(Pepperidge Farm):		
Country Rye	⅒ of loaf	185
White	⅒ of loaf	165
(Rich's):		
French	⅟₂₀ of loaf	138
Italian	⅟₂₀ of loaf	300
Raisin	⅟₂₀ of loaf	107
Wheat	.5-oz. slice	375
White	.8-oz. slice	96
***BREAD MIX** (Pillsbury):		
Applesauce spice	⅟₁₂ of loaf	155
Apricot nut or banana	⅟₁₂ of loaf	150
Blueberry nut	⅟₁₂ of loaf	155
Nut	⅟₁₂ of loaf	180
BROCCOLI:		
Frozen:		
(Birds Eye):		
With cheese sauce	⅓ of 10-oz. pkg.	443
Chopped	⅓ of 10-oz. pkg.	17
Cuts or spears	⅓ of 10-oz. pkg.	20
Spears with hollandaise sauce	⅓ of 10-oz. pkg.	115
(Green Giant):		
In cheese sauce	3⅓ oz.	356
Cuts, polybag	½ cup	13
(McKenzie) chopped or spears	⅓ pkg.	18
(Mrs. Paul's) in cheese sauce	⅓ pkg.	575

Food and Description	Measure or Quantity	Sodium (mgs.)
(Stouffer's) in cheddar cheese sauce	4½ oz.	972
BRUSSELS SPROUT:		
Boiled	3–4 sprouts	8
Frozen:		
(Birds Eye) baby with cheese sauce	⅓ pkg.	361
(Birds Eye) baby, deluxe	⅓ pkg.	5
(Green Giant) in butter sauce	⅓ pkg.	247
(Green Giant) halves in cheese sauce	⅓ pkg.	394
(Kounty Kist)	⅓ pkg.	17
(McKenzie)	3⅓ oz.	12
BUC*WHEATS, cereal (General Mills)	1 oz. (¾ cup)	235
BULGUR, canned, seasoned	4-oz. serving	522
BURGER KING:		
Apple pie	3-oz. pie	335
Cheeseburger	1 burger	730
Cheeseburger, double meat	1 burger	990
French fries	1 regular order	230
Hamburger	1 burger	525
Onion rings	1 regular order	450
Pepsi, diet	1 medium-sized drink	52
Shake:		
Chocolate	1 shake	280
Vanilla	1 shake	340
Whopper:		
Regular	1 burger	990
Regular, with cheese	1 burger	1435
Double beef	1 burger	1080
Double beef, with cheese	1 burger	1535
Junior	1 burger	560
Junior, with cheese	1 burger	785
BURGUNDY WINE:		
(Gold Seal)	3 fl. oz.	3
(Great Western)	3 fl. oz.	36
BURGUNDY WINE, SPARKLING:		
(Gold Seal)	3 fl. oz.	3
(Great Western)	3 fl. oz.	36
BURRITO:		
*Canned (Del Monte)	1 burrito	616
Frozen:		
(Hormel):		
Cheese	1 burrito	448
Hot chili	1 burrito	474

15

Food and Description	Measure or Quantity	Sodium (mgs.)
(Van de Kamp's) & guacamole sauce	6 oz.	652
BURRITO FILLING MIX (Del Monte)	1 cup	1797
BUTTER:		
Salted:		
Regular:		
(Breakstone)	1 T.	95
(Sealtest)	1 T.	117
Whipped (Breakstone)	1 T.	64
Unsalted (Breakstone):		
Regular	1 T.	<1
Whipped	1 T.	<1
BUTTERSCOTCH MORSELS (Nestlé)	1 oz.	21

C

Food and Description	Measure or Quantity	Sodium (mgs.)
CABBAGE:		
Boiled, white, without salt, drained	½ cup (3.2 oz.)	12
Canned (Greenwood's) red, solids & liq.	½ cup	475
Frozen (Green Giant) stuffed	7-oz. serving	823
CAKE:		
Regular, non-frozen:		
Plain, home recipe, with butter, with boiled white icing	⅑ of 9″ square	299
Angel food, home recipe	1/12 of 8″ cake	113
Caramel, home recipe, with caramel icing	⅑ of 9″ square	214
Carrot (Hostess)	3-oz. piece	179
Chocolate, home recipe, with chocolate icing, 2-layer	1/12 of 9″ cake	235
Crumb (Hostess)	1¼-oz. cake	98
Fruit:		
Home recipe, dark	1/30 of 8″ loaf	24
Home recipe, light, made with butter	1/30 of 8″ loaf	29
(Holland Honey Cake) unsalted	1/14 of cake	2

Food and Description	Measure or Quantity	Sodium (mgs.)
Pound, home recipe, traditional, made with butter	3½″ × 3½″ slice	53
Raisin Date Loaf (Holland Honey Cake) low sodium	¹⁄₁₄ of 13-oz. cake	2
Sponge, home recipe	¹⁄₁₂ of 10″ cake	110
White, home recipe, made with butter, without icing, 2-layer	⅑ of 9″ wide, 3″ high cake	279
Yellow, home recipe, made with butter, without icing, 2-layer	¹⁄₁₉ of cake	260
Frozen:		
Apple Walnut:		
(Pepperidge Farm) with cream cheese icing	⅛ of 11¾-oz. cake	140
(Sara Lee)	⅛ of 12½-oz. cake	140
Banana (Sara Lee)	⅛ of 13¾-oz. cake	154
Banana nut (Sara Lee) layer	⅛ of 20-oz. cake	167
Black forest (Sara Lee)	⅛ of 21-oz. cake	140
Boston Cream (Pepperidge Farm)	¼ of 11¾-oz. cake	190
Carrot (Sara Lee)	⅛ of 12¼-oz. cake	125
Cheesecake:		
(Rich's) Viennese	¹⁄₁₄ of 42-oz. cake	298
(Sara Lee):		
Blueberry, *For 2*	½ of 11.3-oz. cake	326
Cherry, *For 2*	½ of 11.3-oz. cake	262
Cream cheese	⅓ of 10-oz. cake	206
Cream cheese, blueberry	⅙ of 19-oz. cake	175
Cream cheese, cherry	⅙ of 19-oz. cake	185
Cream cheese, strawberry	⅙ of 19-oz. cake	170
Chocolate:		
(Pepperidge Farm):		
Layer, Fudge	¹⁄₁₀ of 17-oz. cake	140
Supreme	¼ of 11½-oz. cake	140
(Sara Lee):		
Regular	⅛ of 13¼-oz. cake	168
German	⅛ of 12¼-oz. cake	134
Layer, 'N Cream	⅛ of 18-oz. cake	136
Coffee (Sara Lee):		
Almond	⅛ of 11¾-oz. cake	158
Almond ring	⅛ of 9½-oz. cake	124
Apple	⅛ of 15-oz. cake	208
Apple, *For 2*	½ of 9-oz. cake	502
Blueberry ring	⅛ of 9¾-oz. cake	135
Butter, *For 2*	½ of 6½-oz. cake	391
Maple crunch ring	⅛ of 9¾-oz. cake	131
Pecan	¼ of 6½-oz. cake	184

Food and Description	Measure or Quantity	Sodium (mgs.)
Pecan	⅛ of 11¼-oz. cake	159
Raspberry ring	⅛ of 9¾-oz. cake	120
Streusel, butter	⅛ of 11½-oz. cake	178
Streusel, cinnamon	⅛ of 10.9-oz. cake	156
Crumb (see ROLL OR BUN, Crumb)		
Devil's Food (Pepperidge Farm)	⅒ of 17-oz. cake	135
Golden (Pepperidge Farm)	⅒ of 17-oz. cake	115
Orange (Sara Lee)	⅛ of 13¾-oz. cake	170
Pound (Sara Lee):		
Regular	⅒ of 10¾-oz. cake	104
Chocolate	⅒ of 10¾-oz. cake	134
Family size	1/15 of 16½-oz. cake	106
Homestyle	⅒ of 9½-oz. cake	97
Strawberry cream (Pepperidge Farm) Supreme	1/12 of 24-oz. cake	145
Strawberries 'n cream, layer (Sara Lee)	⅛ of 20½-oz. cake	150
Strawberry Shortcake (Sara Lee)	⅛ of 21-oz. cake	81
Torte (Sara Lee):		
Apples 'n cream	⅛ of 21-oz. cake	146
Fudge & nut	⅛ of 15¾-oz. cake	144
Vanilla (Pepperidge Farm) layer	⅒ of 17-oz. cake	120
Walnut, layer (Sara Lee)	⅛ of 18-oz. cake	102
CAKE OR COOKIE ICING		
(Pillsbury) all flavors	1 T.	5
CAKE ICING:		
Butter pecan (Betty Crocker) *Creamy Deluxe*	1/12 of can	85
Caramel, home recipe	4-oz.	94
Cherry (Betty Crocker) *Creamy Deluxe*	1/12 of can	95
Chocolate:		
(Betty Crocker) *Creamy Deluxe:*		
Regular	1/12 of can	95
Chip	1/12 of can	85
Fudge, dark dutch	1/12 of can	125
Milk	1/12 of can	95
Nut	1/12 of can	95
Sour cream	1/12 of can	110
(Duncan Hines) regular	1/12 of can	84
(Pillsbury) *Frosting Supreme:*		
Fudge	1/12 of can	90
Milk	1/12 of can	50
Sour cream	1/12 of can	90

Food and Description	Measure or Quantity	Sodium (mgs.)
Coconut almond (Pillsbury) *Frosting Supreme*	¹⁄₁₂ of can	60
Cream cheese:		
(Betty Crocker) *Creamy Deluxe*	¹⁄₁₂ of can	100
(Pillsbury) *Frosting Supreme*	¹⁄₁₂ of can	80
Double dutch (Pillsbury) *Frosting Supreme*	¹⁄₁₂ of can	60
Lemon:		
(Betty Crocker) *Sunkist, Creamy Deluxe*	¹⁄₁₂ of can	95
(Pillsbury) *Frosting Supreme*	¹⁄₁₂ of can	45
Orange (Betty Crocker) *Creamy Deluxe*	¹⁄₁₂ of can	95
Strawberry (Pillsbury) *Frosting Supreme*	¹⁄₁₂ of can	45
Vanilla:		
(Betty Crocker) *Creamy Deluxe*	¹⁄₁₂ of can	95
(Duncan Hines)	¹⁄₁₂ of can	86
(Pillsbury) *Frosting Supreme*	¹⁄₁₂ of can	80
White:		
Home recipe, boiled	4 oz.	162
Home recipe, uncooked	4 oz.	56
(Betty Crocker) *Creamy Deluxe*	¹⁄₁₂ of can	95
*CAKE ICING MIX:		
Regular:		
Banana (Betty Crocker) *Chiquita*, creamy	¹⁄₁₂ of pkg.	100
Butter Brickle (Betty Crocker) creamy	¹⁄₁₂ of pkg.	115
Butter pecan (Betty Crocker) creamy	¹⁄₁₂ of pkg.	100
Caramel (Pillsbury) *Rich 'n Easy*	¹⁄₁₂ of pkg.	35
Cherry (Betty Crocker) creamy	¹⁄₁₂ of pkg.	100
Chocolate:		
Home recipe, fudge	½ cup	478
(Betty Crocker) creamy:		
Fluffy, almond fudge, fudge creamy or sour cream	¹⁄₁₂ of pkg.	75
Fudge, dark	¹⁄₁₂ of pkg.	90
Milk	¹⁄₁₂ of pkg.	80
(Pillsbury) *Rich 'N Easy:*		
Fudge	¹⁄₁₂ of pkg.	70
Milk	¹⁄₁₂ of pkg.	55
Coconut almond (Pillsbury)	¹⁄₁₂ of pkg.	85
Coconut pecan:		
(Betty Crocker) creamy	¹⁄₁₂ of pkg.	100

Food and Description	Measure or Quantity	Sodium (mgs.)
(Pillsbury)	1/12 of pkg.	105
Cream cheese & nut (Betty Crocker) creamy	1/12 of pkg.	100
Double dutch (Pillsbury) *Rich 'N Easy*	1/12 of pkg.	80
Lemon:		
(Betty Crocker) *Sunkist*, creamy	1/12 of pkg.	100
(Pillsbury) *Rich 'N Easy*	1/12 of pkg.	15
Strawberry (Pillsbury) *Rich 'N Easy*	1/12 of pkg.	55
Vanilla (Pillsbury) *Rich 'N Easy*	1/12 of pkg.	30
White:		
(Betty Crocker) fluffy	1/12 of pkg.	40
(Betty Crocker) sour cream, creamy	1/12 of pkg.	100
(Pillsbury) fluffy	1/12 of pkg.	65
Dietetic (Betty Crocker) *Lite* chocolate, lemon or vanilla	1/12 of pkg.	50
CAKE MIX:		
Regular:		
Angel Food:		
(Betty Crocker):		
Chocolate or Confetti	1/12 pkg.	275
One-step	1/12 pkg.	250
Strawberry	1/12 pkg.	270
Traditional	1/12 pkg.	140
(Duncan Hines)	1/12 pkg.	119
*(Pillsbury) white	1/12 of cake	345
*Apple Cinnamon (Betty Crocker) *Super Moist*	1/12 of cake	275
Applesauce raisin (Betty Crocker) *Snackin' Cake*	1/9 pkg.	250
*Applesauce spice (Pillsbury) *Pillsbury Plus*	1/12 of cake	300
Banana:		
*(Betty Crocker) *Super Moist*	1/12 of cake	255
*(Pillsbury) *Pillsbury Plus*	1/12 of cake	290
*(Pillsbury) *Streusel Swirl*	1/16 of cake	200
Banana walnut (Betty Crocker) *Snackin' Cake*	1/9 pkg.	260
*Boston cream (Pillsbury) *Bundt*	1/16 of cake	305
*Butter (Pillsbury):		
Pillsbury Plus	1/12 of cake	345
Streusel Swirl, rich	1/16 of cake	235
*Butter Brickle (Betty Crocker) *Super Moist*	1/12 of cake	265

20

Food and Description	Measure or Quantity	Sodium (mgs.)
*Butter pecan (Betty Crocker) *Super Moist*	1/12 of cake	250
*Butter yellow (Betty Crocker) *Super Moist*	1/12 of cake	200
*Carrot (Betty Crocker) *Super Moist*	1/12 of cake	255
Carrot nut (Betty Crocker) *Snackin' Cake*	1/9 of pkg.	240
*Carrot 'n spice (Pillsbury) *Pillsbury Plus*	1/12 of cake	330
*Cheesecake:		
(Jell-O)	1/8 of 8″ cake	306
(Royal)	1/8 of cake	442
*Cherry chip (Betty Crocker) *Super Moist*	1/12 of cake	265
Chocolate:		
(Betty Crocker):		
*Pudding	1/6 of cake	255
Snackin' Cake:		
Almond	1/9 pkg.	215
Fudge chip	1/9 pkg.	205
German, coconut pecan	1/9 pkg.	255
Stir 'N Frost:		
with chocolate frosting	1/6 pkg.	200
Fudge, with vanilla frosting	1/6 pkg.	250
Stir 'N Streusel (Betty Crocker) German	1/6 pkg.	245
Super Moist:		
*Chocolate chip	1/12 of cake	425
*Fudge	1/12 of cake	450
*German	1/12 of cake	420
*Milk	1/12 of cake	290
*Sour cream	1/12 of cake	430
*(Pillsbury):		
Bundt:		
Fudge nut crown	1/16 of cake	290
Fudge, triple	1/16 of cake	330
Fudge, tunnel of	1/16 of cake	315
Macaroon	1/16 of cake	305
Pillsbury Plus:		
Fudge, dark	1/12 of cake	440
Fudge, marble	1/12 of cake	300
German	1/12 of cake	340
Mint	1/12 of cake	340
Streusel Swirl, German	1/16 of cake	290

Food and Description	Measure or Quantity	Sodium (mgs.)
Cinnamon (Betty Crocker) *Stir 'N Streusel*	⅙ of pkg.	230
Coconut pecan (Betty Crocker) *Snackin' Cake*	⅑ of pkg.	255
Coffee cake:		
*(Aunt Jemima)	⅛ of cake	34
*(Pillsbury):		
Apple cinnamon	⅛ of cake	155
Butter pecan	⅛ of cake	335
Cinnamon streusel	⅛ of cake	225
Sour cream	⅛ of cake	235
Date nut (Betty Crocker) *Snackin' Cake*	⅑ of pkg.	265
Devil's food:		
*(Betty Crocker) *Super Moist*	1/12 of cake	425
(Duncan Hines) deluxe	1/12 pkg.	363
*(Pillsbury) *Pillsbury Plus*	1/12 of cake	405
Fudge (See Chocolate)		
Golden chocolate chip (Betty Crocker) *Snackin' Cake*	⅑ of pkg.	255
Lemon:		
(Betty Crocker):		
*Chiffon	1/12 of cake	190
Pudding	⅙ of cake	270
Stir 'N Frost, with lemon frosting	1/12 of pkg.	210
Super Moist	1/12 of cake	260
*(Pillsbury):		
Bundt, tunnel of	1/16 of cake	295
Pillsbury Plus	1/12 of cake	310
Streusel Swirl	1/16 of cake	335
*Lemon blueberry (Pillsbury) *Bundt*	1/16 of cake	270
Marble:		
*(Betty Crocker) *Super Moist*	1/12 of cake	255
*(Pillsbury):		
Bundt, supreme, ring	1/16 of cake	265
Streusel Swirl, fudge	1/16 of cake	200
*Oats 'N brown sugar (Pillsbury) *Pillsbury Plus*	1/12 of cake	300
*Orange (Betty Crocker) *Super Moist*	1/12 of cake	280
Pound:		
*(Betty Crocker) golden	1/12 of cake	155
*(Pillsbury) *Bundt*	1/16 of cake	260

Food and Description	Measure or Quantity	Sodium (mgs.)
Spice (Betty Crocker):		
Snackin' Cake, raisin	⅑ of pkg.	250
Super Moist	¹⁄₁₂ of cake	260
Strawberry:		
(Betty Crocker) Super Moist	¹⁄₁₂ of cake	260
(Pillsbury) Pillsbury Plus	¹⁄₁₂ of cake	300
*Upside down (Betty Crocker)		
pineapple	⅑ of cake	215
White:		
*(Betty Crocker):		
Stir 'N Frost, with chocolate		
frosting	⅙ of cake	235
Super Moist	¹⁄₁₂ of cake	275
(Duncan Hines) deluxe	¹⁄₁₂ of pkg.	251
(Pillsbury) Pillsbury Plus	¹⁄₁₂ of cake	295
Yellow:		
(Betty Crocker) Super Moist	¹⁄₁₂ of cake	270
(Duncan Hines) deluxe	¹⁄₁₂ of pkg.	271
(Pillsbury) Pillsbury Plus	¹⁄₁₂ of cake	300
*Dietetic (Estee)	¹⁄₁₀ of cake	15
CANDY, REGULAR:		
Almond, chocolate covered		
(Hershey's) *Golden Almond*	1 oz.	17
Almond Cluster (Heath)	1 oz.	47
Almond, Jordan	1 oz.	6
Baby Ruth	1.8-oz. piece	102
Breath Saver (Life Saver)	1 piece	TR.
Butter Brickle Bar (Heath)	1 oz.	73
Butterfinger	1.6-oz. bar	68
Caramel:		
Caramel Nip (Pearson)	1 piece	34
Caramel Pattie (Heath)	1-oz. serving	56
Cereal Raisin Bar (Heath)	2-oz. serving	76
Chocolate bar:		
Choco-Lite (Nestlé)	.27-oz. bar	5
Choco-Lite (Nestlé)	1-oz. serving	18
Crunch (Nestlé)	¹⁄₁₆-oz. bar	57
Krunch (Heath)	1½-oz. serving	100
Milk:		
(Heath) crunch with toffee	2¼-oz. serving	108
(Heath) solid	2¼-oz. serving	71
(Hershey's)	1.2-oz. bar	31
(Hershey's)	4-oz. bar	102
(Nestlé)	.35-oz. bar	8
(Nestlé)	¹⁄₁₆-oz. bar	24
Special Dark (Hershey's)	1.05-oz. bar	<1

Food and Description	Measure or Quantity	Sodium (mgs.)
Special Dark (Hershey's)	4-oz. bar	3
Chocolate bar with almonds:		
(Heath)	2½-oz. serving	79
(Hershey's) milk	.35-oz. bar	8
(Hershey's) milk	1.15-oz. bar	26
(Hershey's) milk	4-oz. bar	91
(Nestlé)	1-oz. serving	20
Chocolate Parfait (Pearson)	1 piece	3
Coffee Nip (Pearson)	1 piece	17
Coffioca (Pearson)	1 piece	5
Gum drops	1 oz.	10
Jelly beans	1 oz.	3
Kisses (Hershey's)	1 piece (.2 oz.)	4
Kit Kat	.6-oz. bar	16
Kit Kat	1⅛-oz. bar	36
Krackel Bar	.35-oz. bar	16
Krackel Bar	1.2-oz. bar	55
Krackel Bar	4-oz. bar	182
Licorice:		
Licorice Nips (Pearson)	1 piece	34
Lollipops (Life Savers)	.9-oz. pop	7
Lollipops (Life Savers)	.6-oz. pop	<5
Mars Bar (M&M/Mars)	1½-oz. serving	62
Marshmallow	1 oz.	11
Mary Jane (Miller):		
Small size	¼ oz.	4
Large size	1½ oz.	23
Milky Way (M&M/Mars)	.8-oz. bar	48
Milky Way (M&M/Mars)	1.9-oz. serving	113
Meltaway (Heath)	1 oz.	22
Mighty Mint (Life Savers)	1 piece	TR.
Mint Parfait (Pearson)	1 piece	5
M & M's:		
Peanut	1½ oz.	25
Plain	1½ oz.	38
Mr. Goodbar (Hershey's)	.35-oz. bar	6
Mr. Goodbar (Hershey's)	1½-oz. bar	26
Mr. Goodbar (Hershey's)	4-oz. bar	68
$100,000 Bar (Nestlé)	1¼-oz. bar	64
Peanut butter cup (Reese's)	.6-oz. cup	41
Reggie Bar	2-oz. bar	40
Rolo (Hershey's)	1 piece	13
Royals, mint chocolate (M&M/Mars)	1½-oz. serving	36
Snickers	1.8-oz. bar	129
Starburst (M&M/Mars)	1.9-oz. serving	13

24

Food and Description	Measure or Quantity	Sodium (mgs.)
Summit, cookie bar (M&M/Mars)	1-oz. serving	41
3 Muskateers	.8-oz. bar	48
3 Muskateers	2-oz. serving	124
Toffee Brickle (Heath)	1 oz.	84
Tootsie Roll:		
Chocolate	.23-oz. midgee	1
Chocolate	⅟₁₆-oz. bar	4
Chocolate	¾-oz. bar	5
Chocolate	1-oz. bar	6
Chocolate	1¾-oz. bar	11
Flavored	.6-oz. square	1
Pop, all flavors	.49-oz. pop	4
Pop drop, all flavors	4.7-gram piece	1
Twix, cookie bar (M&M/Mars)	1¾-oz. serving	95
Twix, peanut butter cookie bar (M&M/Mars)	1¾-oz. serving	159
Whatchamacallit (Hershey's)	1.15-oz. bar	75
CANDY, DIETETIC:		
Carob bar, *Joan's Natural:*		
Coconut	1 section of 3-oz. bar	10
Coconut	3-oz. bar	117
Fruit & nut	1 section of 3-oz.bar	10
Fruit & nut	3-oz. bar	115
Honey bran	1 section of 3-oz. bar	9
Honey bran	3-oz. bar	114
Peanut	1 section of 3-oz. bar	9
Peanut	3-oz. bar	109
Chocolate or chocolate flavored bar (Estee):		
Bittersweet	1 section of 2½-oz. bar	3
Bittersweet	2½-oz. bar	42
Coconut	1 section of 2½-oz. bar	5
Coconut	2½-oz. bar	61
Crunch	1 section of 2-oz. bar	5
Crunch	2-oz. bar	65
Fruit & nut	1 section of 2½-oz. bar	5
Fruit & nut	2½-oz. bar	59
Milk	1 section of 2½-oz. bar	6
Milk	2½-oz. bar	68
Toasted bran	1 section of 2½-oz. bar	5.1
Toasted bran	2½-oz. bar	62

Food and Description	Measure or Quantity	Sodium (mgs.)
Chocolate bar with almonds (Estee) milk	1 section of 2½-oz. bar	5
Chocolate bar with almonds (Estee) milk	2½-oz. bar	61
Estee-etts, with peanuts (Estee)	1 piece	<1
Gum drops (Estee) any flavor	1 piece	<1
Peanut butter cup (Estee)	1 cup	8
Raisins, chocolate-covered (Estee)	1 piece	1
T.V. mix (Estee)	1 piece	2
CANNELLONI FLORENTINE, frozen (Weight Watchers) one-compartment	13-oz. meal	894
CANTALOUPE, cubed	½ cup	10
CAP'N CRUNCH, cereal (Quaker):		
Regular	¾ cup	185
Crunchberry	¾ cup	166
Peanut butter	¾ cup	210
CARAWAY SEED (French's)	1 tsp.	<1
CARNATION INSTANT BREAKFAST:		
Bar:		
Chocolate Chip	1 bar	163
Chocolate Crunch	1 bar	129
Peanut Butter Crunch	1 bar	154
Dry:		
Chocolate or chocolate malt	1 packet	187
Coffee	1 packet	130
Strawberry	1 packet	194
Vanilla	1 packet	145
CARROT:		
Raw	5½" × 1" carrot	24
Boiled, sliced	½ cup	23
Canned, regular:		
(Del Monte) drained	½ cup	336
(Libby's) solids & liq.	½ cup	280
(Stokely-Van Camp) solids & liq.	½ cup	263
Canned, dietetic:		
(Featherweight) solids & liq.	½ cup	30
(S&W) *Nutradiet*, sliced, solids & liq.	½ cup	50
Frozen:		
(Birds Eye) with brown sugar glaze	⅓ pkg.	503
(Green Giant) cuts in butter sauce	⅓ pkg.	315
(McKenzie)	⅓ pkg.	44

Food and Description	Measure or Quantity	Sodium (mgs.)
CASABA MELON	1-lb. melon	27
CASHEW NUT:		
(Fisher):		
Dry roasted	1 oz.	57
Oil roasted	1 oz.	78
(Planters):		
Dry roasted, salted	1 oz.	222
Oil roasted, salted	1 oz.	219
CATSUP:		
Regular:		
(Del Monte)	1 T.	181
(Smucker's)	1 T.	107
Dietetic:		
(Featherweight)	1 T.	5
(Tillie Lewis) *Tasti Diet*	1 T.	6
CAULIFLOWER:		
Raw or boiled buds	½ cup	6
Frozen:		
(Birds Eye)	⅓ pkg.	16
(Green Giant) in cheese sauce	⅓ pkg.	377
(McKenzie)	3⅓ oz.	16
(Mrs. Paul's) light batter & cheese	⅓ pkg.	650
(Stouffer's) in cheddar cheese sauce	4½ oz.	776
CAVIAR, whole eggs	1 T.	352
CELERY:		
1 large outer stalk	8″ × 1½″ at root end	50
Diced or cut	½ cup	67
Salt (French's)	1 tsp.	1505
Seed (French's)	1 tsp.	4
CHABLIS WINE (Great Western)	3 fl. oz.	31
CHAMPAGNE (Great Western)	3 fl. oz.	31
CHARLOTTE RUSSE, homemade recipe	4 oz.	49
CHEERIOS, cereal (General Mills):		
Regular	1¼ cups	330
Honey-Nut	¾ cup	255
CHEESE:		
American or cheddar:		
Cube, natural	1″ cube	119
(Featherweight) low sodium	1 oz.	6
(Sargento):		
Midget, regular or sharp	1 oz.	176
Shredded, non-dairy	1 oz.	269
Blue:		
(Frigo)	1 oz.	511

27

Food and Description	Measure or Quantity	Sodium (mgs.)
(Sargento) cold pack or crumbled	1 oz.	396
Brick (Sargento)	1 oz.	159
Brie (Sargento) *Danish Danko*	1 oz.	282
Burgercheese (Sargento)	1 oz.	406
Camembert (Sargento) *Danish Danko*	1 oz.	233
Colby:		
(Featherweight) low sodium	1 oz.	4
(Sargento) shredded or sliced	1 oz.	171
Cottage:		
Unflavored:		
(USDA)	1 oz.	65
(Friendship) no salt added	1 oz.	8
Cream, plain, unwhipped:		
(USDA)	1 oz.	71
Philadelphia (Kraft)	1 oz.	113
Edam:		
(House of Gold)	1 oz.	204
(Sargento)	1 oz.	274
Farmers:		
(Friendship) no salt added	1 oz.	2
(Sargento)	1 oz.	132
Feta (Sargento) Danish, cups	1 oz.	316
Gjetost (Sargento) Norwegian	1 oz.	170
Gouda:		
(Sargento) baby, caraway or smoked	1 oz.	232
Wispride	1 oz.	298
Gruyere, *Swiss Knight*	1 oz.	362
Havarti (Sargento), creamy or creamy, 60% mild	1 oz.	198
Hot pepper (Sargento)	1 oz.	171
Jarlsberg (Sargento) Norwegian	1 oz.	130
Kettle Moraine (Sargento)	1 oz.	17
Limburger (Sargento) natural	1 oz.	227
Monterey Jack:		
(Frigo)	1 oz.	204
(Sargento) Midget, Longhorn, shredded or sliced	1 oz.	152
Mozzarella:		
(Frigo) part skim milk	1 oz.	227
(Sargento):		
Bar, rounds, shredded, shredded with spices, sliced for pizza or square	1 oz.	150

Food and Description	Measure or Quantity	Sodium (mgs.)
Whole milk	1 oz.	106
Muenster:		
(Sargento) red rind	1 oz.	178
Wispride	1 oz.	129
Nibblin Curds (Sargento)	1 oz.	176
Parmesan:		
(Frigo):		
Grated	1 T.	88
Whole	1 oz.	341
(Sargento), wedge	1 oz.	454
Pizza (Sargento) shredded or sliced	1 oz.	306
Pot (Sargento) regular, French onion or garlic	1 oz.	<1
Provolone:		
(Frigo)	1 oz.	284
(Sargento) sliced	1 oz.	248
Ricotta (Sargento):		
Part skim milk	1 oz.	35
Whole milk	1 oz.	24
Romano (Sargento) wedge	1 oz.	340
Roquefort, natural	1 oz.	460
Samsoe (Sargento) Danish	1 oz.	198
Scamorze (Frigo)	1 oz.	227
String (Sargento)	1 oz.	150
Swiss:		
(USDA) natural	1 oz.	201
(Sargento) domestic, or Finland, sliced	1 oz.	74
Taco (Sargento) shredded	1 oz.	47
CHEESE FONDUE, *Swiss Knight*	1-oz. serving	186
CHEESE FOOD:		
American or cheddar:		
(Weight Watchers) colored or white	1-oz. slice	533
Wispride:		
Regular	1 oz.	205
& blue cheese	1 oz.	265
Hickory smoked	1 oz.	233
& port wine	1 oz.	253
Cheez 'N Crackers (Kraft)	1 piece	466
Cheez-ola (Fisher)	1 oz.	454
Cracker Snack (Sargento)	1 oz.	406
Mun-chee (Pauly)	1 oz.	485
Pimiento (Pauly)	.8-oz. slice	426
Swiss (Pauly)	.8-oz. slice	58

Food and Description	Measure or Quantity	Sodium (mgs.)
CHEESE SOUFFLE, home recipe	¼ of 7" souffle (3.9 oz.)	400
CHEESE SPREAD:		
American or cheddar:		
(Nabisco) *Snack Mate*	1 tsp.	65
Cheese 'n Bacon (Nabisco) *Snack Mate*	1 tsp.	58
Cheez Whiz (Kraft)	1 oz.	473
Count Down (Fisher)	1 oz.	439
Imitation (Fisher) *Chef's Delight*	1 oz.	380
Pimiento:		
(Nabisco) *Snack Mate*	1 tsp.	60
(Price's)	1 oz.	335
Sharp (Pauly)	.8 oz.	437
Swiss, process (Pauly)	.8 oz.	391
Velveeta (Kraft)	1 oz.	431
CHERRY, sweet:		
Fresh, with stems	½ cup	1
Canned, regular (Stokley-Van Camp) pitted, solids & liq.	½ cup	18
Canned, dietetic, solids & liq.:		
(Diet Delight) with pits, water pack	½ cup	5
(Featherweight) dark, water pack	½ cup	<10
(Featherweight) light, water pack	½ cup	<1.0
CHERRY DRINK (Hi-C):		
Canned	6 fl. oz.	4
*Mix	6 fl. oz.	23
CHERRY JELLY:		
Sweetened (Smucker's)	1 T.	3
Dietetic:		
(Featherweight)	1 T.	45
(Slenderella)	1 T.	22
CHERRY PRESERVE OR JAM:		
Sweetened (Smucker's)	1 T.	6
Dietetic, (Featherweight) imitation	1 T.	45
CHESTNUT, fresh, in shell	¼ lb.	7
CHEWING GUM:		
Sweetened:		
Beechies	1 piece	<1
Doublemint, Freedent or *Juicy Fruit*	1 piece	TR.
CHEX, cereal (Ralston Purina):		
Corn	1 cup	295
Rice	1 cup	243

30

Food and Description	Measure or Quantity	Sodium (mgs.)
Wheat	⅔ cup	192
Wheat & raisins	¾ cup	216
CHICKEN:		
Broiler, cooked, meat only	3 oz.	56
Fryer, fried, meat & skin	3 oz.	66
Fryer, fried, meat only	3 oz.	66
Fryer, fried, a 2½ lb. chicken (weighed with bone before cooking) will give you:		
Dark meat with skin	4 oz.	100
Light meat with skin	4 oz.	77
Hen & cock:		
Stewed, dark meat only	3 oz.	55
Stewed, light meat only	3 oz.	41
Stewed, diced	½ cup	37
Roaster, roasted, dark or light meat without skin	3 oz.	65
CHICKEN À LA KING:		
Home recipe	1 cup	760
Canned (Swanson)	½ of 10½-oz. can	710
Frozen:		
(Banquet) *Cookin' Bag*	5-oz. pkg.	892
(Stouffer's) with rice	9½ oz.	900
(Weight Watchers)	10-oz. bag	1273
CHICKEN BOUILLON:		
(Herb-Ox):		
Cube	1 cube	950
Packet	1 packet	960
(Maggi)	1 cube	699
Low sodium (Featherweight)	1 tsp.	5
CHICKEN, BONED, CANNED:		
(Swanson) chunk:		
Regular	2½ oz.	340
Mixin chicken	2½ oz.	280
White	2½ oz.	240
Low sodium (Featherweight)	2½ oz.	49
CHICKEN DINNER OR ENTREE:		
Canned (Swanson) & dumplings	7½ oz.	980
Frozen:		
(Banquet):		
Regular:		
& dumplings	12-oz. dinner	1914
Fried	11-oz. dinner	2371
Nuggets	12-oz. entree	674
Buffet Supper	2-lb. pkg.	5190

Food and Description	Measure or Quantity	Sodium (mgs.)
Man-Pleaser		
& dressing	19-oz. dinner	1807
& dumpling	19-oz. dinner	1814
Fried	17-oz. dinner	2477
(Green Giant):		
& broccoli with rice in cheese sauce	10-oz. entree	1034
& pea pods in sauce with rice & vegetables	10-oz. entree	1026
(Morton):		
Boneless	10-oz. dinner	1457
Country Table, fried	12-oz. entree	614
(Stouffer's):		
Cacciatore	11¼ oz.	1135
Divan	8½ oz.	830
Papribash	10½ oz.	1325
(Swanson):		
Regular, in white wine sauce	8¼-oz. entree	845
Hungry Man:		
Boneless	19-oz. dinner	1575
Fried:		
Dark portion with whipped potatoes	10¼-oz. entree	1235
TV Brand, fried:		
Barbecue	11¼-oz. dinner	850
Nibbles	6-oz. entree	750
With whipped potatoes	7¼-oz. entree	1110
White portions	11½-oz. dinner	1395
3-course, fried	15-oz. dinner	1715
(Weight Watchers):		
New Orleans style	11-oz. bag	1132
Oriental style	12-oz. bag	1596
Parmigiana, 2-compartment	7¾-oz. pkg.	1030
Sliced, in celery sauce, 2-compartment	8½-oz. pkg.	925
Sliced with gravy & stuffing, 3-compartment	14¾-oz. pkg.	1915
Sweet & sour	9½-oz. bag	563
CHICKEN, FRIED, frozen:		
(Banquet)	2-lb. bag	6518
(Morton)	2-lb. pkg.	7909
(Swanson):		
Assorted pieces	3.2-oz. serving	705
Breast	3.2-oz. serving	620
Nibbles (wing)	3.2-oz. serving	645
Take-out style	4-oz. serving	730

Food and Description	Measure or Quantity	Sodium (mgs.)
Thighs & drumsticks	3.2-oz. serving	625
CHICKEN LIVER & Onion, frozen (Weight Watchers) 2-compartment	9¼-oz. meal	497
CHICKEN & NOODLES:		
Frozen:		
(Banquet) *Buffet Supper*	2-lb. pkg.	5645
(Green Giant) with vegetables	9-oz. pkg.	371
CHICKEN PIE, frozen:		
(Banquet)	8-oz. pie	999
(Stouffer's)	10-oz. pie	1530
(Swanson)		
Regular	8-oz. pie	810
Hungry Man	1-lb. pie	1680
(Van de Kamp's)	7½-oz. pie	890
CHICKEN SALAD (Carnation)	1½-oz. serving	230
CHICKEN SOUP (See SOUP, Chicken)		
CHICKEN SPREAD:		
(Swanson)	1-oz. serving	230
(Underwood)	1-oz. serving	240
CHICKEN STEW, canned:		
Regular:		
(Bounty)	7½-oz. serving	1022
(Libby's) with dumplings	8-oz. serving	976
(Swanson)	7⅝-oz. serving	960
Dietetic:		
(Dia-Mel)	8-oz. can	65
(Featherweight)	7¼-oz. can	53
CHICKEN STOCK BASE (French's)	1 tsp.	475
CHICK PEAS OR GARBANZOS, dry	¼ lb.	29
CHILI OR CHILI CON CARNE:		
Canned, regular pack:		
Beans only (Van Camp) Mexican style	1 cup	900
With beans:		
(Libby's)	½ of 15-oz. can	810
(Swanson)	7¾-oz. sering	1100
Without beans (Libby's)	7½ oz.	1182
Canned, dietetic pack (Featherweight) with beans	7½-oz.	85
Frozen, with beans (Weight Watchers) one-compartment	10-oz. pkg.	822
CHILI SAUCE:		
(Ortega) green	1 oz.	175
(Featherweight) dietetic	1 T.	10

Food and Description	Measure or Quantity	Sodium (mgs.)
CHILI SEASONING MIX:		
*(Durkee)	1 cup	979
(French's) *Chili-O*	1 pkg.	3780
CHOCO-DILE (Hostess)	2-oz. piece	284
CHOCOLATE, BAKING:		
(Baker's):		
Bitter or unsweetened	1 oz.	1
Semi-sweet, chips	¼ cup	9
Sweetened, *German's*	1 oz.	<1
(Hershey's):		
Bitter or unsweetened	1 oz.	<1
Sweetened:		
Dark, chips, regular or mini	1 oz.	65
Milk, chips	1 oz.	37
Semi-sweet, chips	1 oz.	3
(Nestlé):		
Bitter or unsweetened, *Choco-Bake*	1-oz. packet	<5
Sweet or semi-sweet, morsels	1 oz.	3
CHOP SUEY, frozen, (Banquet) beef:		
Buffet Supper	2-lb. pkg.	5336
Cookin' Bag	7-oz. bag	1140
Dinner	12-oz. dinner	1802
***CHOP SUEY** SEASONING MIX*		
(Durkee)	1¾ cups	5582
CHOWDER (See SOUP, Chowder)		
CHOW CHOW:		
Sour	1 oz.	379
Sweet	1 oz.	149
CHOW MEIN:		
Canned:		
(Chun King) chicken	8-oz. serving	924
(La Choy):		
Beef	1 cup	977
*Beef, bi-pack	1 cup	1009
Chicken	½ of 1-lb. can	924
*Chicken, bi-pack	1 cup	928
Meatless	1 cup	835
*Mushroom, bi-pack	1 cup	1161
Pepper Oriental	1 cup	1024
*Pepper Oriental, bi-pack	1 cup	1559
*Pork, bi-pack	1 cup	1625
Shrimp	1 cup	951
*Shrimp, bi-pack	1 cup	1079
Frozen:		
(Banquet)	12-oz. dinner	2268

34

Food and Description	Measure or Quantity	Sodium (mgs.)
(Green Giant) chicken	9-oz. entree	1076
(La Choy):		
Beef, 5-compartment	11-oz. dinner	5912
Beef, entree	8-oz. serving	1226
(Stouffer's) chicken	8 oz.	1115
CINNAMON, GROUND (French's)	1 tsp.	<1
CITRUS COOLER DRINK, canned (Hi-C)	6 fl. oz.	4
CLAM:		
Raw, all kinds, meat only	1 cup (8 oz.)	466
Frozen (Mrs. Paul's):		
Deviled	3-oz. piece	682
Fried	2½ oz.	675
CLAMATO COCKTAIL (Mott's)	6 fl. oz.	815
CLAM CHOWDER (See CHOWDER, Clam)		
CLARET WINE (Gold Seal)	3 fl. oz.	3
CLOVES (French's)	1 tsp.	4
COCOA:		
Dry, unsweetened (Hershey's)	1 T.	<1
Mix, regular:		
(Alba '66) instant, all flavors	1 envelope	89
(Carnation) all flavors	1-oz. pkg.	115
(Hershey's):		
Hot	1 oz.	142
Instant	3 T.	36
(Nestlé):		
Hot	1 oz.	188
With mini marshmallows	1 oz.	159
(Ovaltine) hot 'n rich	1-oz. pkg.	183
Swiss Miss regular or with mini marshmallows	6 fl. oz.	110
Mix, dietetic:		
(Carnation) *70 Calorie*	¾-oz. packet	125
(Ovaltine) hot, reduced calorie	.45-oz. pkg.	88
COCOA KRISPIES, cereal (Kellogg's)	¾ cup	195
COCOA PUFFS, cereal (General Mills)	1 oz. (1 cup)	205
COCONUT:		
Fresh, meat only	2″ × 2″ × ½″ piece	10
Grated or shredded, loosely packed	½ cup	15
Dried:		
(Baker's):		
Angel Flake	⅓ cup	64

Food and Description	Measure or Quantity	Sodium (mgs.)
Cookie	⅓ cup	87
Premium shred	⅓ cup	74
(Durkee) shredded	¼ cup	5
COCO WHEATS, cereal	1 T.	3
COD, broiled	3 oz.	94
COFFEE:		
Regular:		
*Max-Pax; Maxwell House Electra Perk, Yuban; Yuban Electra Matic, Mellow Roast	6 fl. oz.	<1
Decaffeinated:		
Brim, regular or	6 fl. oz.	5
Decaf; Nescafé; Taster's Choice	6 fl. oz.	<10
Sanka, regular or electric perk	6 fl. oz.	TR.
*Freeze-dried, *Maxim, Sanka, Taster's Choice*	6 fl. oz.	TR.
Instant:		
*(Chase & Sanborn)	5 fl. oz.	1
Decaf (Nestlé); *Nescafé; Sunrise*	6 fl. oz.	<10
*Mellow Roast	6 fl. oz.	2
*Mix (General Foods) *International Coffee:*		
Cafe Amaretto; Cafe Francais; Irish Mocha Mint; Suisse Mocha	6 fl. oz.	25
Cafe Vienna	6 fl. oz.	93
Orange Cappucino	6 fl. oz.	98
COFFEE CAKE (See CAKE, Coffee)		
COFFEE SOUTHERN	1 fl. oz.	TR.
COLA SOFT DRINK (See SOFT DRINK, Cola)		
COLD DUCK WINE (Great Western) pink	3 fl. oz.	31
COLESLAW, solids & liq., made with mayonnaise-type salad dressing	1 cup	148
COLLARDS:		
Leaves & stems, boiled	½ cup	28
Canned (Sunshine) chipped, solids & liq.	½ cup	378
Frozen:		
(Birds Eye) chopped	⅓ pkg.	45
(McKenzie) chopped	3⅓ oz.	45
COMPLETE CEREAL (Elam's)	1 oz.	5
CONCORD WINE:		
(Gold Seal)	3 fl. oz.	3
(Peasant Valley) red	3 fl. oz.	23
COOKIE, REGULAR:		

Food and Description	Measure or Quantity	Sodium (mgs.)
Animal:		
(Dixie Belle)	1 piece	7
(Nabisco) *Barnum's Animals*	1 piece	12
(Ralston)	1 piece	7
Apple (Pepperidge Farm)	1 piece	26
Apple Spice (Pepperidge Farm)	1 piece	26
Apricot Raspberry (Pepperidge Farm)	1 piece	26
Assortment (Pepperidge Farm):		
Butter	1 piece	27
Champagne & Original Pirouette	1 piece	18
Chocolate Laced Pirouette	1 piece	15
Marseilles & Seville	1 piece	25
Southport	1 piece	35
Bordeaux (Pepperidge Farm)	1 piece	23
Brown edge wafers (Nabisco)	1 piece	20
Brownie:		
(Frito-Lays) nut fudge	1.8-oz. piece	146
(Hostess)	1¼-oz. piece	76
(Pepperidge Farm) chocolate nut	.4-oz. piece	27
(Sara Lee) frozen	⅛ of 13-oz. pkg.	108
Brussels (Pepperidge Farm)	1 piece	32
Butter (Nabisco)	1 piece	17
Cappucino (Pepperidge Farm)	1 piece	20
Capri (Pepperidge Farm)	1 piece	45
Chessmen (Pepperidge Farm)	1 piece	26
Chocolate & chocolate-covered:		
(Nabisco):		
Pinwheel, cake	1 piece	30
Snap	1 piece	14
Chocolate chip:		
(Nabisco) *Chips Ahoy!*	1 piece	31
(Pepperidge Farm)		
Regular	1 piece	30
Large	1 piece	80
Chocolate	1 piece	25
Cinnamon Sugar (Pepperidge Farm)	1 piece	53
Coconut Granola (Pepperidge Farm)	1 piece	27
Creme Stick (Dutch Twin)		
chocolate coated	1 piece	3
Date Nut Granola (Pepperidge Farm)	1 piece	32
Date Pecan (Pepperidge Farm)	1 piece	53
Devil's food cake (Nabisco)	1 piece	31
Fig bar	1 oz. (1⅝" sq.)	71
Fig Newtons (Nabisco)	1 piece	53
Geneva (Pepperidge Farm)	1 piece	21
Gingerman (Pepperidge Farm)	1 piece	25

Food and Description	Measure or Quantity	Sodium (mgs.)
Gingersnaps (Nabisco) old fashioned	1 piece	41
Granola (Pepperidge Farm)	1 piece	85
Hazelnut (Pepperidge Farm)	1 piece	37
Ladyfinger	3¼″ × ⅜″ × 1⅛″	8
Lemon Nut (Pepperidge Farm)	1 piece	60
Lido (Pepperidge Farm)	1 piece	42
Macaroon, coconut (Nabisco)	1 piece	29
Marshmallow:		
(Nabisco):		
Mallomars	1 piece	19
Puffs, cocoa covered	1 piece	25
Sandwich	1 piece	22
Twirls cakes	1 piece	32
Milano (Pepperidge Farm)	1 piece	26
Mint Milano (Pepperidge Farm)	1 piece	35
Molasses Crisp (Pepperidge Farm)	1 piece	25
Nassau (Pepperidge Farm)	1 piece	45
Nilla wafer (Nabisco)	1 piece	12
Oatmeal:		
(Keebler) old fashion	1 piece	76
(Pepperidge Farm):		
Irish	1 piece	40
Large	1 piece	105
Raisin	1 piece	57
Orange Milano (Pepperidge Farm)	1 piece	35
Orleans (Pepperidge Farm)	1 piece	10
Peanut & peanut butter:		
(Nabisco) *Nutter Butter*	1 piece	57
(Pepperidge Farm) chip:		
Regular	1 piece	45
Large	1 piece	110
Pecan Sandies (Keebler)	1 piece	52
Raisin	1 oz.	15
Raisin (Nabisco) fruit biscuit	1 piece	19
Raisin Bran (Pepperidge Farm)	1 piece	27
Sandwich:		
(Nabisco):		
Mystic mint	1 piece	46
Oreo	1 piece	49
Shortbread or shortcake		
(Nabisco):		
Lorna Doone	1 piece	39
Pecan	1 piece	44
Social Tea, biscuit (Nabisco)	1 piece	18
Spiced wafers (Nabisco)	1 piece	58
St. Moritz (Pepperidge Farm)	1 piece	23

Food and Description	Measure or Quantity	Sodium (mgs.)
Sugar cookie (Nabisco) rings, *Bakers Bonus*	1 piece	47
Sugar wafer:		
(Dutch Twin)	1 piece	2
(Keebler) *Krisp Kreem*	1 piece	14
(Nabisco) *Biscos*	1 piece	5
Sunflower Raisin (Pepperidge Farm)	1 piece	25
Tahiti (Pepperidge Farm)	1 piece	25
Vanilla creme (Wise)	1 piece	23
Vanilla wafer (Keebler)	1 piece	18
Zanzibar (Pepperidge Farm)	1 piece	13
COOKIE, DIETETIC (Estee)	1 piece	<1
COOKIE CRISP, cereal (Ralston Purina):		
Chocolate chip	1 cup	188
Vanilla wafer	1 cup	200
COOKIE DOUGH:		
Refrigerated (Pillsbury):		
Chocolate chip or Oatmeal	1 cookie	42
Peanut Butter	1 cookie	73
Frozen (Rich's):		
Chocolate chip	1 cookie	120
Oatmeal	1 cookie	90
Sugar	1 cookie	111
COOKIE MIX:		
Regular:		
Brownie:		
(Betty Crocker):		
Fudge, regular size	¹⁄₁₆ of pan	100
Walnut, family size	¹⁄₂₄ of pan	85
(Duncan Hines)	¹⁄₂₄ of pan	88
(Pillsbury) fudge, regular size	1½" square (¹⁄₃₆ of pan)	43
Chocolate chip:		
(Betty Crocker) *Big Batch*	1 cookie	47
(Duncan Hines)	¹⁄₃₆ of pkg.	42
(Quaker)	1 cookie	70
Date bar (Betty Crocker)	¹⁄₃₂ of pkg.	35
Macaroon, coconut (Betty Crocker)	¹⁄₂₄ of pkg.	15
Oatmeal:		
(Betty Crocker) *Big Batch*	1 cookie	50
(Duncan Hines) raisin	¹⁄₃₆ of pkg.	31
(Nestlé) raisin	1 cookie	43
(Quaker)	1 cookie	71
Peanut butter (Duncan Hines)	1 cookie	57

Food and Description	Measure or Quantity	Sodium (mgs.)
Sugar:		
(Betty Crocker) *Big Batch*	1 cookie	47
(Duncan Hines) golden	1/36 of pkg.	33
Dietetic (Dia-Mel)	2" cookie	20
CORN:		
Fresh, on the cob, boiled	5" × 1¾" ear	TR.
Canned, regular pack:		
(Del Monte):		
Cream style, golden, wet pack	½ cup	411
Whole kernel, drained	½ cup	285
Whole Kernel, vacuum pack	½ cup	233
(Festal):		
Cream style, golden, wet pack	½ cup	411
Golden, whole kernel, drained	½ cup	285
(Green Giant):		
Cream style	4¼ oz.	321
Whole kernel, solids & liq.	4¼ oz.	297
Whole kernel, *Mexicorn*, solids & liq.	3½ oz.	288
(Libby's):		
Cream style	½ cup	295
Whole kernel, solids & liq.	½ cup	264
(Stokely-Van Camp):		
Cream style	½ cup	383
Whole kernel, solids & liq.	½ cup	290
Canned, dietetic pack:		
(Diet Delight) solids & liq.	½ cup	5
(Featherweight) whole kernel, solids & liq.	½ cup	<10
(S&W) *Nutradiet*, solids & liq.	½ cup	<10
Frozen:		
(Birds Eye):		
On the cob, *Farmside*	4.4-oz. ear	3
On the cob, *Little Ears*	2.3-oz. ear	2
Jubilee	⅓ of pkg.	264
Whole kernel	⅓ of pkg.	3
(Green Giant):		
On the cob	5½" ear	1
On the cob, *Nibbler*	3" ear	<1
Whole kernel, *Harvest Fresh*	4 oz.	278
Whole kernel, *Niblets*, golden, in butter sauce	⅓ of pkg.	235
Whole kernel, white, in butter sauce	⅓ of pkg.	243
(McKenzie) on the cob	5" ear	4

Food and Description	Measure or Quantity	Sodium (mgs.)
CORNBREAD:		
Home recipe:		
Corn pone	4 oz.	449
Spoon bread	4 oz.	547
*Mix:		
(Aunt Jemima)	⅙ of pkg.	600
(Pillsbury) *Ballard*	⅛ of recipe	570
***CORN DOGS**, frozen (Oscar Mayer)	4-oz. piece	1282
CORNED BEEF:		
Cooked, boneless, medium fat	4 oz.	1973
Canned:		
Dinty Moore	3-oz. serving	895
(Libby's)	⅓ of 7-oz. can	720
Dietetic (Featherweight) loaf	2½ oz.	53
Packaged (Oscar Mayer) jellied loaf	1-oz. slice	285
CORNED BEEF HASH, canned:		
(Libby's)	1 cup (8 oz.)	1330
Mary Kitchen	7½-oz. serving	1481
CORNED BEEF HASH DINNER, frozen (Banquet)	10-oz. dinner	1752
CORNED BEEF SPREAD (Underwood)	1 oz.	269
CORN FLAKE CRUMBS (Kellogg's)	¼ cup	305
CORN FLAKES, cereal:		
(Featherweight) low sodium	1 cup	10
(General Mills) *Country*	1 cup	310
(Kellogg's)	1 cup	285
(Kellogg's) honey & nut	¾ cup	190
(Post) *Post Toasties*	1¼ cups	299
(Ralston Purina):		
Regular	1 cup	267
Sugar frosted	¾ cup	179
(Van Brode) low sodium	1 cup	2
CORN MEAL:		
Bolted	¼ cup	TR.
Degermed	¼ cup	TR.
Mix, bolted (Aunt Jemima) self-rising	1 cup	2292
CORNSTARCH (Argo; Kingsford's; Duryea)	1 tsp.	TR.
CORN SYRUP (See SYRUP)		
COUGH DROP:		
(Beech-Nut)	1 drop	<1
(Pine Bros.)	1 drop	<1

Food and Description	Measure or Quantity	Sodium (mgs.)
COUNT CHOCULA, cereal (General Mills)	1 oz. 1 cup	205
CRAB APPLE, flesh only	¼ lb.	1
CRAB APPLE JELLY (Smucker's)	1 T.	3
CRAB, DEVILED, breaded & fried (Mrs. Paul's) regular	½ of 6-oz. pkg.	510
CRAB IMPERIAL, home recipe	1 cup	1602
CRACKER, PUFFS & CHIPS:		
American Harvest (Nabisco)	1 piece	36
Arrowroot biscuit (Nabisco)	1 piece	11
Bacon Nips	1 oz.	700
Bran Wafer (Featherweight)	1 piece	<1
Bugles (General Mills)	1 oz.	285
Cheese flavored:		
Cheddar Bitz (Frito-Lay)	1 oz.	239
Cheese filled (Frito-Lay's)	1½ oz.	383
Chee-Tos, crunchy	1 oz.	290
Chee-Tos, puffed	1 oz.	470
Cheez Balls (Planters)	1 oz.	301
Cheez Curls (Planters)	1 oz.	301
Curl (Featherweight)	1 oz.	81
(Dixie Belle)	1 piece	10
(Ralston)	1 piece	10
Tid-Bit (Nabisco)	1 oz.	15
Chicken in a Biskit (Nabisco)	1 piece	19
Chippers (Nabisco)	1 piece	48
Chipsters (Nabisco)	1 piece	8
Club cracker (Keebler)	1 piece	44
Corn chip:		
(Featherweight)	1 oz.	3
Fritos	1 oz.	204
Fritos, barbecue flavor	1 oz.	270
Korkers (Nabisco)	1 piece	11
Corn Nuggets (Frito-Lay's)	1 oz.	264
Crown Pilot (Nabisco)	1 piece	64
Doo Dads (Nabisco)	1 piece	7
English Water Biscuit (Pepperidge Farm)	1 piece	24
Escort (Nabisco)	1 piece	37
Flings (Nabisco)	1 piece	16
French onion cracker (Nabisco)	1 piece	31
Goldfish (Pepperidge Farm):		
Thins:		
Butter Flavor	1 piece	12
Cheese or lightly salted	1 piece	15

Food and Description	Measure or Quantity	Sodium (mgs.)
Tiny:		
Cheddar cheese, lightly salted, pizza or pretzel	1 piece	4
Parmesan	1 piece	6
Graham:		
(Dixie Belle) sugar-honey coated	1 piece	26
Honey Maid (Nabisco)	1 piece	52
(Nabisco)	1 piece	44
Graham, chocolate or cocoa-covered:		
Fancy Dip (Nabisco)	1 piece	41
(Keebler)	1 piece	27
(Nabisco)	1 piece	34
Onion Toast (Keebler)	1 piece	29
Oyster:		
(Keebler) *Zesta*	1 piece	4
(Nabisco) *Dandy or Oysterettes*	1 piece	11
Ritz (Nabisco)	1 piece	32
Roman Meal Wafer, boxed	1 piece	20
Rye Toast (Keebler)	1 piece	39
Ry-Krisp, natural	1 triple cracker	48
Ry-Krisp, seasoned	1 triple cracker	65
Saltine:		
(Dixie Belle) unsalted	1 piece	21
Premium (Nabisco)	1 piece	35
Zesta (Keebler)	1 piece	34
Sea Toast (Keebler)	1 piece	112
Sesame:		
Butter flavored (Nabisco)	1 piece	35
Snackers (Ralston)	1 piece	23
Snackin' Crisp (Durkee) *O & C*	1 oz.	257
Snacks Sticks (Pepperidge Farm):		
Cheese or sesame	1 piece	43
Lightly salted	1 piece	40
Parmesan Nutzel	1 piece	24
Pumpernickel or Rye	1 piece	48
Tortillo chips:		
Doritos, nacho or taco flavor	1 oz.	108
(Planters) nacho or taco flavor	1 oz.	170
Unsalted (Featherweight)	2 sections (½ cracker)	1
Wheat (Pepperidge Farm) cracked	1 piece	52
Wheat Snack (Ralston)	1 piece	12
Wheat Wafer (Featherweight) unsalted	1 piece	<1
CRACKER CRUMBS, graham	1 cup (not packed)	576
CRACKER MEAL	1 T.	110

Food and Description	Measure or Quantity	Sodium (mgs.)
CRANAPPLE JUICE (Ocean Spray)		
canned:		
Regular	6 fl. oz.	4
Dietetic	6 fl. oz.	8
CRANBERRY, fresh (Ocean Spray)	½ cup	<1
***CRANBERRY JUICE COCKTAIL**		
canned (Ocean Spray):		
Regular	6 fl. oz.	3
Dietetic	6 fl. oz.	6
CRANBERRY-ORANGE RELISH		
(Ocean Spray)	1 T.	5
CRANBERRY-RASPBERRY		
SAUCE (Ocean Spray) jellied	2-oz. serving	14
CRANBERRY SAUCE:		
Home recipe	4 oz.	1
canned (Ocean Spray):		
Jellied	2-oz. serving	17
Whole berry	2-oz. serving	16
CRANGRAPE (Ocean Spray)	6 fl. oz.	5
CRAZY COW, cereal (General Mills)	1 cup	185
CREAM:		
Half & Half	1 T.	7
Light, table or coffee (Sealtest) 16% fat	1 T.	6
Light, whipping, 30% fat (Sealtest)	1 T.	5
Heavy whipping, unwhipped	1 T.	5
Sour	1 T.	5
Substitute (See CREAM SUBSTITUTE)		
CREAM PUFFS:		
Home recipe, custard filling	3½″ × 2″ piece	108
Frozen (Rich's) chocolate	1⅓ oz. piece	83
CREAM SUBSTITUTE:		
Coffee Mate (Carnation)	1 tsp.	4
Coffee Rich	½ oz.	7
N-Rich	1½ tsp.	17
CREME DE MENTHE (Leroux) green	1 fl. oz.	<1
CREPE, frozen:		
(Mrs. Paul's):		
Crab	5½ oz.	1156
Shrimp	5½ oz.	1046
(Stouffer's):		
Beef burgundy	6¼ oz.	830
Chicken with mushroom sauce	8½ oz.	1040
Ham & swiss cheese	7½ oz.	905
Spinach	9½ oz.	995

44

Food and Description	Measure or Quantity	Sodium (mgs.)
Swiss cheese with mustard sauce	8⅜ oz.	955
CRESS, GARDEN, raw, whole	1 lb.	45
CRISP RICE, cereal:		
(Featherweight) low sodium	1 cup	<10
(Ralston Purina)	1 cup	206
(Van Brode) low sodium	1 cup	2
CRISPY WHEATS 'N RAISINS, cereal (General Mills)	¾ cup	180
CROQUETTES, frozen, seafood (Mrs. Paul's)	3-oz. serving	869
CROUTON:		
(Kellogg's) *Croutettes*	⅔ cup	260
(Pepperidge Farm):		
Cheddar & romano or sour cream & chive	.5 oz.	185
Cheese & garlic	.5 oz.	175
Seasoned	.5 oz.	215
CUCUMBER:		
Eaten with skin	½-lb. cucumber	13
Pared, 10-oz. cucumber	7½" × 2" pared	12
Pared	3 slices	1
CUMIN SEED (French's)	1 tsp.	3
CUPCAKE:		
Regular (Hostess):		
Chocolate	1 cupcake	249
Orange	1 cupcake	170
Frozen (Sara Lee) yellow	1 cupcake	161
*CUPCAKE MIX** (Flako)	1 cupcake	195
CURRANT, dried, Zante (Del Monte)	½ cup	4
CURRANT JELLY (Smucker's)	1 T.	7
CUSTARD:		
Chilled, *Swiss Miss*, egg flavor	4-oz. container	180
*Mix, dietetic (Featherweight)	½ cup	105
C. W. POST, cereal:		
Plain	¼ cup	49
With raisins	¼ cup	44

D

DAIRY QUEEN/BRAZIER:

Banana split	13.5-oz. serving	153
Brownie Delight, hot fudge	9.4-oz. serving	227
Buster Bar	5¼-oz. piece	179
Chicken sandwich	7.76-oz. sandwich	869
Cone:		
Plain, any flavor:		
Small	3-oz. cone	47
Regular	5-oz. cone	78
Large	7½-oz. cone	117
Dipped, chocolate:		
Small	3¼-oz. cone	55
Regular	5½-oz. cone	94
Large	8¼-oz. cone	140
Dilly Bar	3-oz. piece	51
Double Delight	9-oz. service†	153
DQ sandwich	2.1-oz. serving	39
Fish sandwich:		
Plain	6-oz. sandwich	875
With cheese	6.24-oz. sandwich	1035
Float	14-oz. serving	79
Freeze, vanilla	14-oz. serving	179
French fries:		
Regular	2½-oz. serving	114
Large	4-oz. serving	181
Frozen dessert	4-oz. serving	62
Hamburger:		
Plain:		
Single	5.2-oz. sandwich	630
Double	7.4-oz. sandwich	660
Triple	9.6-oz. sandwich	690
With cheese:		
Single	5.7-oz. sandwich	790
Double	8.43-oz. sandwich	980
Triple	10.62-oz. sandwich	1010

46

Food and Description	Measure or Quantity	Sodium (mgs.)
Hot dog:		
Regular:		
Plain	3.53-oz. serving	830
With cheese	4-oz. serving	990
With chili	4½-oz. serving	985
Super:		
Plain	6.2-oz. serving	1365
With cheese	6.9-oz. serving	1605
With chili	7.7-oz. serving	1595
Lettuce	½ oz.	<10
Malt, chocolate:		
Small	10.26-oz. serving	180
Regular	14.74-oz. serving	260
Large	20.74-oz. serving	360
Mr. Misty:		
Plain:		
Small	8¾-oz. serving	<10
Regular	11.64-oz. serving	<10
Large	15.5-oz. serving	<10
Kiss	3.14-oz. serving	<10
Float	14½-oz. serving	95
Freeze	14½-oz. serving	140
Onion rings	3-oz.	140
Parfait	10 oz.	140
Peanut Butter Parfait	10¾-oz. serving	250
Shake, chocolate:		
Small	10¼-oz. serving	180
Regular	14¾-oz. serving	260
Large	20¾-oz. serving	360
Strawberry shortcake	11 oz.	215
Sundae, chocolate:		
Small	3¾-oz. serving	75
Regular	6¼-oz. serving	120
Large	8¾-oz. serving	165
Tomato	½ oz.	<10
DATE, domestic:		
Chopped	½ cup	1
Pitted	4 oz.	1
DELI'S, frozen (Pepperidge Farm):		
Beef with barbecue sauce	4 oz.	685
Mexican style	4 oz.	645
Reuben in rye pastry	4 oz.	650
Turkey, ham & cheese	4 oz.	740
Western style omelet	4 oz.	555
DESSERT CUPS (Hostess)	¾-oz. piece	119
DILL SEED (French's)	1 tsp.	TR.

Food and Description	Measure or Quantity	Sodium (mgs.)
DING DONG (Hostess)	1 cake	132
DINNER, frozen (See individual listings such as BEEF, CHICKEN, TURKEY, etc.)		
DIP:		
Blue cheese (Dean) tang	1 oz.	14
Enchilada, *Fritos*	1 oz.	97
Jalapeno, *Fritos*	1 oz.	88
Onion (Dean) French	1 oz.	20
DISTILLED LIQUOR, any brand	1 fl. oz.	<1
DONUTZ, cereal (General Mills):		
Chocolate	1-oz. piece	210
Powdered	1-oz. piece	185
DOUGHNUT (See also **WINCHELL'S**):		
Regular (Hostess):		
Chocolate coated	1-oz. piece	151
Cinnamon	1-oz. piece	111
Crunch	1-oz. piece	134
Donnettes, frosted or powdered	1 piece	51
Old fashioned	1½-oz. piece	217
Old fashioned, glazed	2-oz. piece	199
Plain	1-oz. piece	135
Powdered	1-oz. piece	153
Frozen (Morton):		
Bavarian creme	2-oz. piece	80
Boston creme	2.3-oz. piece	93
Chocolate iced	1½-oz. piece	77
Glazed	1½-oz. piece	72
Jelly	1.8-oz. piece	78
Mini	1.1-oz. piece	204
DRUMSTICK, frozen:		
Ice cream, in a cone:		
Topped with peanuts	1 piece	82
Topped with peanuts & cone bisque	1 piece	72
Ice milk, in a cone:		
Topped with peanuts	1 piece	87
Topped with peanuts & cone bisque	1 piece	77
DUMPLINGS, canned, dietetic (Featherweight)	7½ oz.	117

E

Food and Description	Measure or Quantity	Sodium (mgs.)
ECLAIR:		
Home recipe, with custard filling and chocolate icing	4-oz. piece	93
Frozen (Rich's) chocolate	1 piece	194
EGG, CHICKEN:		
Raw, white only	1 large egg	48
Raw, yolk only	1 large egg	9
Boiled	1 large egg	61
Fried in butter	1 large egg	155
Omelet, mixed with milk & cooked in fat	1 large egg	159
Poached	1 large egg	130
Scrambled, mixed with milk & cooked in fat	1 large egg	164
EGG MIX (Durkee):		
Omelet:		
*With bacon	½ of pkg.	276
*Puffy	½ of pkg.	333
Scrambled:		
Plain	.8-oz. pkg.	320
With bacon	1.3-oz. pkg.	476
EGG NOG, dairy (Sealtest) 6% fat	½ cup	80
EGGPLANT:		
Boiled	4 oz.	1
Frozen:		
(Mrs. Paul's):		
Parmesan	5½-oz. serving	1100
Slices, breaded & fried	3-oz. serving	660
Sticks, breaded & fried	3½-oz. serving	875
(Weight Watchers) parmigiana	13-oz. pkg.	1073
EGG ROLL, frozen (La Choy):		
Chicken	.4-oz. roll	66
Lobster	.4-oz. roll	62
Meat & shrimp	.2-oz. roll	43
Meat & shrimp	.4-oz. roll	81
Shrimp	.4-oz. roll	64

Food and Description	Measure or Quantity	Sodium (mgs.)
Shrimp	2½-oz. roll	393
EGG, SCRAMBLED, frozen (Swanson) and sausage with hashed brown potatoes, TV Brand	6½-oz. entree	730
EGG SUBSTITUTE:		
Egg Magic (Featherweight)	½ envelope	123
Scramblers (Morningstar Farms)	1 egg	63
Second Nature (Avoset)	3 T.	68
ELDERBERRY JELLY (Smucker's)	1 T.	TR.
ENCHILADA, frozen:		
Beef:		
(Banquet):		
Buffet Supper, with cheese & chili gravy	2-lb. pkg.	6336
Dinner	12-oz. dinner	2326
(Green Giant) Sonora style	12-oz. entree	1251
(Swanson) *TV Brand*	15-oz. dinner	1575
(Van de Kamp's):		
Dinner	12-oz. dinner	2177
Entree, shredded	12-oz. entree	1296
Cheese:		
(Banquet) *Man-Pleaser*	21¼-oz. dinner	2510
(Van de Kamp's)	12-oz. dinner	1664
Chicken (Van de Kamp's)	7½-oz. pkg.	1108
ENCHILADA SAUCE:		
Canned (Del Monte) hot	½ cup	1151
*Mix (Durkee)	½ cup	48
ENDIVE, CURLY OR ESCAROLE, cut up	½ cup	5

F

FARINA:		
(Hi-O) dry, regular	¼ cup	2
Malt-O-Meal, dry, regular	1 oz.	3
Malt-O-Meal, dry, quick cooking	1 oz.	2
*(Pillsbury) made with milk & salt	⅔ cup	480
FAT, COOKING	1 T.	0
FENNEL SEED (French's)	1 tsp.	2

Food and Description	Measure or Quantity	Sodium (mgs.)
FETTUCINI ALFREDO, frozen		
(Stouffer's)	5 oz.	1194
FIG:		
Small	1½" fig	<1
Canned, regular pack (Del Monte)		
whole solids & liq.	½ cup	1
Dried, chopped	½ cup	29
FIGURINES (Pillsbury):		
Caramel nut	1 bar	110
Chocolate	1 bar	75
Chocolate mint	1 bar	80
Lemon yogurt	1 bar	60
Vanilla	1 bar	72
FILBERT:		
Shelled	1 oz.	<1
(Fisher) oil dipped, salted	½ cup	114
FISH CAKE, frozen (Mrs. Paul's)		
thins, breaded & fried	½ of 10-oz. pkg.	1850
FISH & CHIPS, frozen:		
(Mrs. Paul's) batter fried, light	½ of 14-oz. pkg.	1050
(Swanson) *TV Brand*	5-oz. entree	570
(Van de Kamp's) batter dipped,		
french fried	8-oz. serving	551
FISH DINNER, frozen:		
(Banquet)	8¾-oz. dinner	1473
(Mrs. Paul's):		
Au gratin	½ of 10-oz. pkg.	850
Parmesan	½ of 10-oz. pkg.	1000
(Van de Kamp's) batter dipped,		
french fried, fillet	12-oz. dinner	1822
(Weight Watchers) in lemon sauce,		
3-compartment	13¼-oz. meal	975
FISH FILLET, frozen:		
(Mrs. Paul's):		
Batter fried, crunchy	2¼-oz. piece	675
Breaded & fried	2-oz. piece	760
Buttered	2½-oz. piece	600
Miniature, batter fried	3-oz. serving	540
(Van de Kamp's):		
Batter dipped, french fried	3-oz. piece	352
Country seasoned	2.4-oz. piece	334
FISH KABOBS, frozen:		
(Mrs. Paul's) light batter	⅓ pkg.	429
(Van de Kamp's):		
Batter dipped	.4-oz. piece	58
Country seasoned	.4-oz. piece	49

Food and Description	Measure or Quantity	Sodium (mgs.)
FISH SEASONING (Featherweight)	¼ tsp.	<1
FISH STICK, frozen:		
(Mrs. Paul's):		
Batter fried	1 stick	149
Breaded & fried	1 stick	135
(Van de Kamp's) batter dipped, french fried	1-oz. piece	154
FIT 'N FROSTY (Alba '77):		
Chocolate	1 envelope	93
Strawberry	1 envelope	115
Vanilla	1 envelope	108
FIVE ALIVE (Snow Crop)	6 fl. oz.	1
FLOUNDER:		
Baked	4 oz.	269
Frozen:		
(Mrs. Paul's) fillets, breaded & fried	2-oz. fillet	380
(Mrs. Paul's) with lemon butter	4¼-oz. serving	808
(Weight Watchers) with lemon flavored bread crumbs	6½-oz. serving	815
(Weight Watchers) in Newburgh sauce	12½-oz. pkg.	784
FLOUR:		
(Aunt Jemima) self-rising	¼ cup	368
Ballard, self-rising	¼ cup	392
Bisquick (Betty Crocker)	¼ cup	350
(Elam's):		
Brown rice, whole grain	¼ cup	2
Buckwheat, pure	¼ cup	1
Pastry	1 oz.	2
Rye, whole grain	¼ cup	2
Soy	1 oz.	4
Gold Medal (Betty Crocker) all-purpose of high protein	¼ cup	<2
La Pina	¼ cup	<2
Pillsbury's Best:		
All-purpose	¼ cup	<1
Rye, medium	¼ cup	1
Sauce & gravy	2 T.	2
Self-rising	¼ cup	392
Presto, self-rising	¼ cup	322
Wondra	¼ cup	<3
FOOD STICKS (Pillsbury) chocolate	1 stick	29
*FRANKEN*BERRY*, cereal (General Mills)	1 cup	205

Food and Description	Measure or Quantity	Sodium (mgs.)
FRANKFURTER:		
(Oscar Mayer):		
Beef	1.6-oz. frankfurter	466
Little Wiener	2" frankfurter	103
Wiener	1.6-oz. frankfurter	514
Wiener, with cheese	1.6-oz. frankfurter	551
(Oscherwitz):		
Regular	1.6-oz. frankfurter	709
Beef	1.5-oz. frankfurter	665
Cocktail	.3-oz. frankfurter	133
Dinner	2.7-oz. frankfurter	1196
Mild	1.5-oz. frankfurter	665
(Swift)	1.6-oz. frankfurter	509
FRENCH TOAST, frozen:		
(Aunt Jemima):		
Regular	1½-oz. slice	216
Cinnamon swirl	1 slice	179
(Swanson) with sausage, *TV Brand*	4½-oz. breakfast	665
FRITTERS, frozen (Mrs. Paul's):		
Apple	2-oz. piece	540
Clam	1.9-oz. piece	342
Corn	2-oz. piece	760
Shrimp	½ of 7¾ oz. pkg.	760
FROOT LOOPS, cereal (Kellogg's)	1 cup	125
FROSTED RICE, cereal (Kellogg's)	1 cup	205
FRUIT BITS, dried (Sun-Maid)	2-oz. serving	24
FRUIT COCKTAIL:		
Canned, regular pack, solids & liq.:		
(Del Monte) regular and chunky	½ cup	5
(Libby's)	½ cup	8
(Stokely-Van Camp)	½ cup	15
Canned, dietetic pack, solids & liq.:		
(Del Monte) *Lite*	½ cup	5
(Diet Delight) syrup or water pack	½ cup	5
(Featherweight) juice or water pack	½ cup	<10
(Libby's) water pack	½ cup	10
FRUIT CUP (Del Monte):		
Mixed fruits	5-oz. container	6
Peaches, diced	5-oz. container	9
FRUIT & FIBER, cereal (Post):		
Apples & cinnamon	½ cup	195
Dates, raisins & walnuts	½ cup	170
FRUIT, MIXED:		
Canned (Del Monte) *Lite*	½ cup	5

Food and Description	Measure or Quantity	Sodium (mgs.)
Frozen (Birds Eye)	5-oz. serving	4
FRUIT PUNCH:		
Canned:		
Capri Sun	6¾ fl. oz.	1
(Hi-C)	6 fl. oz.	<1
Chilled:		
Five Alive (Snow Crop)	6 fl. oz.	1
(Minute Maid)	6 fl. oz.	<1
*Frozen, *Five Alive* (Snow Crop)	6 fl. oz.	1
*Mix (Hi-C)	6 fl. oz.	1
FRUIT ROLL, frozen (La Choy)	.5-oz. roll	3
FRUIT ROLL-UPS (Betty Crocker)	1 roll	5
FRUIT SALAD:		
Canned, regular pack:		
(Del Monte) fruits for salad	½ cup	4
(Libby's)	½ cup	8
Canned, dietetic pack:		
(Diet Delight)	½ cup	5
(Featherweight) juice or water pack	½ cup	<10
FRUIT SQUARES, frozen (Pepperidge Farm):		
Apple	2½-oz. piece	175
Blueberry	2½-oz. piece	190
Cherry	2½-oz. piece	185

G

GARLIC:		
Flakes (Gilroy)	1 tsp.	<1
Powder (French's)	1 tsp.	<1
Salt (French's)	1 tsp.	1850
GEFILTE FISH, canned (Rokeach) jellied, whitefish & pike	4 oz.	835
***GELATIN DESSERT MIX:**		
Regular (Jell-O):		
Apricot, black cherry, mixed fruit, orange, peach, raspberry, strawberry or strawberry-banana	½ cup	55

Food and Description	Measure or Quantity	Sodium (mgs.)
Cherry	½ cup	77
Lemon or wild strawberry	½ cup	81
Dietetic:		
Carmel Kosher	½ cup	<10
(D-Zerta) all flavors	½ cup	9
(Featherweight) artificially sweetened	½ cup	2
GERMAN STYLE DINNER		
(Swanson) *TV Brand*	11¾-oz. dinner	668
GINGER, powder (French's)	1 tsp.	<1
***GINGERBREAD MIX:**		
(Betty Crocker)	⅑ of cake	325
(Pillsbury)	3″ square	310
***GOLDEN GRAHAMS**, cereal		
(General Mills)	1 cup	285
***GRAHAM CRAKOS**, cereal		
(Kellogg's)	1 cup	145
GRANOLA BARS, *Nature Valley*:		
Almond or peanut	1 bar (.8 oz.)	80
Cinnamon or oats 'n honey	1 bar (.65 oz.)	51
Cinnamon, coconut or oats 'n honey	1 bar (.8 oz.)	65
***GRANOLA BAR MIX** Nature Valley Bake-A-Bar*:		
Chocolate chip	1 bar	40
Peanut butter	1 bar	60
GRANOLA CEREAL, *Nature Valley*	⅓ cup	35
GRANOLA CLUSTERS, *Nature Valley*:		
Almond	1 roll	140
Apple-cinnamon	1 roll	125
Caramel	1 roll	95
GRANOLA & FRUIT BAR, *Nature Valley*:		
Apple or raspberry	1 bar	150
Date	1 bar	135
GRAPE:		
American ripe (slipskin)	3½″ × 3″ bunch	2
Canned, dietetic (Featherweight) light, seedless, water pack	½ cup	<10
GRAPE DRINK:		
Canned:		
Capri Sun	6¾ fl. oz.	19
(Hi-C)	6 fl. oz.	<1
*Mix (Hi-C)	6 fl. oz.	42

Food and Description	Measure or Quantity	Sodium (mgs.)
GRAPEFRUIT:		
Pink & red:		
Seeded type	½ med. grapefruit	1
Seedless type	½ med. grapefruit	1
White:		
Seeded type	½ med. grapefruit	1
Seedless type	½ med. grapefruit	1
Canned, regular pack (Del Monte) in syrup	½ cup	2
Canned, dietetic pack, solids & liq.:		
(Del Monte) sections	½ cup	2
(Diet Delight) sections	½ cup	5
(Featherweight) sections, juice pack	½ cup	<10
GRAPEFRUIT JUICE:		
Fresh, pink, red or white	½ cup	1
Canned, sweetened:		
(Del Monte)	6 fl. oz.	2
(Minute Maid)	6 fl. oz.	2
Canned, unsweetened:		
(Del Monte)	6 fl. oz.	2
(Libby's)	6 fl. oz.	5
(Ocean Spray)	6 fl. oz.	7
(Texsun)	6 fl. oz.	2
Chilled (Minute Maid)	6 fl. oz.	2
*Frozen (Minute Maid)	6 fl. oz.	<1
GRAPEFRUIT JUICE COCKTAIL, canned (Ocean Spray) pink	6 fl. oz.	15
GRAPE JAM (Smucker's)	1 T.	5
GRAPE JELLY:		
Sweetened (Smucker's)	1 T.	6
Dietetic (See GRAPE SPREAD)		
GRAPE JUICE:		
Canned, Unsweetened:		
(Seneca Foods)	6 fl. oz.	4
(Welch's)	6 fl. oz.	<10
*Frozen (Minute Maid)	6 fl. oz.	2
GRAPE NUTS, cereal:		
Regular	¼ cup	197
Flakes	⅞ cup	218
GRAPE SPREAD, dietetic:		
(Diet Delight)	1 T.	3.0
(Estee)	1 T.	TR.
(Featherweight)	1 T.	45
GRAVY, canned:		
Au jus (Franco-American)	2-oz. serving	370

Food and Description	Measure or Quantity	Sodium (mgs.)
Beef (Franco-American)	2-oz. serving	330
Brown:		
(Franco-American) with onion	2-oz. serving	340
(La Choy)	5-oz. can	1111
Ready Gravy	¼ cup	<2
Chicken (Franco-American)	2-oz. serving	320
Mushroom (Franco-American)	2-oz. serving	320
Turkey (Franco-American)	2-oz. serving	300
GRAVYMASTER	1 tsp.	<1
GRAVY WITH MEAT OR TURKEY:		
Canned (Morton House):		
Sliced beef	6¼-oz. serving	1076
Sliced turkey	6¼-oz. serving	995
Frozen:		
(Banquet):		
Giblet gravy & sliced turkey, *Cookin' Bag*	5-oz. bag	836
Sliced beef, *Buffet Supper*	2-lb. pkg.	5381
(Swanson) sliced beef with whipped potatoes, *TV Brand*	8-oz. entree	805
GRAVY MIX:		
Regular:		
Au jus:		
*(Durkee)	½ cup	457
*(French's) *Gravy Makins*	½ cup	530
Brown:		
*(Durkee):		
Regular	½ cup	519
With onions	½ cup	678
*(French's) *Gravy Makins*	½ cup	560
*(Pillsbury)	½ cup	610
Chicken:		
(Durkee):		
*Regular	½ cup	855
*Creamy	½ cup	764
Roastin' Bag	1½-oz. pkg.	3597
*(French's) *Gravy Makins*	½ cup	600
*(Pillsbury)	½ cup	460
Home style:		
*(Durkee)	½ cup	415
*(French's) *Gravy Makins*	½ cup	670
*(Pillsbury)	½ cup	600
Meatloaf (Durkee) *Roastin' Bag*	1½-oz. pkg.	3472
Mushroom:		
*(Durkee)	½ cup	565

Food and Description	Measure or Quantity	Sodium (mgs.)
*(French's) *Gravy Makins*	½ cup	610
Onion:		
*(Durkee)	½ cup	476
*(French's) *Gravy Makins*	½ cup	700
Pork:		
*(Durkee)	½ cup	1087
*(French's) *Gravy Makins*	½ cup	560
*Swiss steak (Durkee)	½ cup	741
Turkey:		
*(Durkee)	½ cup	663
*(French's) *Gravy Makins*	½ cup	768
Dietetic (Weight Watchers):		
Brown	1 pkg.	1339
Brown, with mushrooms	1 pkg.	1495
Brown, with onion	1 pkg.	1475
Chicken	1 pkg.	2087
GREENS, MIXED, canned (Sunshine) solids & liq.	½ cup	468
GUAVA	1 guava	3
GUAVA NECTAR (Libby's)	6 fl. oz.	5

H

HADDOCK:		
Fried, breaded	4″ × 3″ × ½″ fillet	177
Frozen:		
(Banquet)	8¾-oz. dinner	1770
(Mrs. Paul's) breaded & fried	2-oz. fillet	560
(Swanson) filet almondine	7½-oz. entree	1044
(Van de Kamp's) batter dipped, french fried	2-oz. piece	265
(Weight Watchers) with stuffing, 2-compartment	7-oz. pkg.	549
HALIBUT:		
Broiled	4″ × 3″ × ½″ steak	168
Frozen (Van de Kamp's) batter dipped, french fried	½ of 8-oz. pkg.	618
HAM:		
Canned:		
(Hormel) chunk	6¾-oz. serving	2075

Food and Description	Measure or Quantity	Sodium (mgs.)
(Oscar Mayer), *Jubilee*, extra lean, cooked	1-oz. serving	346
(Swift):		
Hostess	3½-oz. slice	1231
Premium	1¾-oz. slice	535
Deviled (Underwood)	1 T.	142
Packaged:		
(Hormel):		
Chopped	1-oz. slice	364
Cooked	.8-oz. slice	266
(Oscar Mayer):		
Chopped	1-oz. slice	378
Cooked, smoked	¾-oz. slice	295
Cooked, smoked	1-oz. slice	399
Jubilee, slice, boneless	8-oz. slice	3029
Jubilee, steak, boneless, 95% fat free	2-oz. steak	739
HAMBURGER (See *McDONALD'S, BURGER KING, DAIRY QUEEN, WHITE CASTLE,* etc.)		
*HAMBURGER MIX, *Hamburger Helper* (General Mills):		
Beef noodle	⅕ of pkg.	970
Beef romanoff	⅕ of pkg.	1095
Cheeseburger	⅕ of pkg.	1025
Hash	⅕ of pkg.	920
Lasagna	⅕ of pkg.	1000
Potatoes au gratin	⅕ of pkg.	890
Potatoes stroganoff	⅕ of pkg.	965
Rice oriental	⅕ of pkg.	1085
Stew	⅕ of pkg.	945
HAMBURGER SEASONING MIX:		
*(Durkee)	1 cup	1012
(French's)	1-oz. pkg.	1700
HAM & CHEESE (Oscar Mayer) loaf	1-oz. serving	370
HAM DINNER, frozen:		
(Banquet)	10-oz. dinner	1590
(Swanson) *TV Brand*	10¼-oz. dinner	1250
HAM SALAD, canned (Carnation)	1½-oz. serving	263
HAM SALAD SPREAD (Oscar Mayer)	1 oz.	259
HEADCHEESE (Oscar Mayer)	1-oz. serving	357
HERRING, SMOKED, hard	4-oz. serving	7066
HO-HO (Hostess)	1-oz. cake	85

Food and Description	Measure or Quantity	Sodium (mgs.)
HOMINY GRITS:		
Dry:		
(Aunt Jemima)	3 T.	1
(Quaker):		
Regular	3 T.	1
Instant:		
Regular	.8-oz. packet	385
With imitation bacon or ham	1-oz. packet	544
With imitation cheese flavor	1oz. packet	497
Cooked	1 cup	502
HONEY, strained	1 T.	1
HONEYCOMB, cereal (Post)	1⅓ cups	214
HONEYDEW	2″ × 7″ wedge	11
HORSERADISH:		
Raw, pared	1 oz.	2
Prepared	1-oz. serving	27
HOSTESS O's (Hostess)	2¼-oz. piece	428

I

ICE CREAM:		
Bar (Heath) *Butter Brickle*	2½-fl. oz. piece	38
Chocolate (Swift's)	½ cup	53
Vanilla (Swift's)	½ cup	52
ICE CREAM CONE, cone only	1 piece	12
*ICE CREAM MIX (Salada):		
Dutch chocolate	1 cup	75
Peach, vanilla or wild strawberry	1 cup	60
ICE MILK:		
Hardened	¼ pt.	44
Soft-serve	¼ pt.	59
ITALIAN DINNER, frozen		
(Banquet)	11-oz. dinner	2156

Food and Description	Measure or Quantity	Sodium (mgs.)

J

JELL-O PUDDING POPS:
  Banana, butterscotch or vanilla | 2-oz. pop | 63
  Chocolate or chocolate fudge | 2-oz. pop | 103
JELLY, sweetened | 1 T. | 3

K

KABOOM, cereal (General Mills)	1 cup	370
KALE:		
Boiled, leaves only	4 oz.	49
Canned (Sunshine) chopped, solids & liq.	½ cup	251
Frozen:		
(Birds Eye) chopped	⅓ of pkg.	14
(McKenzie) chopped	⅓ of pkg.	14
KIDNEY:		
Beef, braised	4 oz.	287
Lamb, raw	4 oz.	257
KING VITAMIN, cereal (Quaker)	1¼ cups	251
KIX, cereal	1½ cups	315
KNOCKWURST (Best's Kosher, Oscherwitz):		
Regular	3-oz. piece	1329
Beef	3-oz. piece	1329
***KOOL-AID** (General Foods):		
Unsweetened (sugar to be added)	8 fl. oz.	0
Pre-sweetened:		
All flavors except tropical punch	8 fl. oz.	Tr.
Tropical punch	8 fl. oz.	10
KUMQUAT, flesh & skin	5 oz.	8

L

LAMB:
Leg:
    Roasted, lean & fat | 3 oz. | 59

Food and Description	Measure or Quantity	Sodium (mgs.)
LAMB:		
Leg:		
Roasted, lean & fat	3 oz.	59
Roasted, lean only	3 oz.	59
Loin, one 5-oz. chop (weighed with cone before cooking) will give you:		
Lean & fat	2.8 oz.	55
Lean only	2.3 oz.	46
Rib, one 5-oz. chop (weighed with bone before cooking) will give you:		
Lean & fat	2.9 oz.	57
Lean only	2 oz.	39
Shoulder:		
Roasted, lean & fat	3 oz.	59
Roasted, lean only	3 oz.	59
LASAGNA:		
Frozen:		
(Green Giant):		
Baked:		
Regular, with meat sauce	12-oz. entree	1595
Chicken	12-oz. entree	1220
Boil 'N Bag	9-oz. entree	1120
(Stouffer's)	10½ oz.	1200
(Swanson):		
Regular, with meat in tomato sauce	13¼-oz. entree	1160
Hungry Man, with meat	17¾-oz. dinner	1487
TV Brand	13-oz. dinner	780
(Weight Watchers)	12¾-oz. meal	869
LEEKS	4 oz.	6
LEMON:		
Whole	2⅛" lemon	3
Peeled	2⅛" lemon	1
LEMONADE:		
Canned:		
Capri Sun	6¾ fl. oz.	2

Food and Description	Measure or Quantity	Sodium (mgs.)
Country Time	6 fl. oz.	58
(Hi-C)	6 fl. oz.	6
Chilled (Minute Maid) regular or pink	6 fl. oz.	<1
*Frozen:		
Country Time regular or pink	6 fl. oz.	11
Minute Maid	6 fl. oz.	<1
*Mix:		
Country Time, regular or pink or lemon-lime	6 fl. oz.	12
Kool Aid, sweetened, regular or pink	6 fl. oz.	<1
(Minute Maid) regular or pink	6 fl. oz.	6
LEMON JUICE:		
Canned, *ReaLemon*	1 T.	<1
*Frozen (Minute Maid) unsweetened	1 fl. oz.	<1
***LEMON-LIMEADE,** mix (Minute Maid)	6 fl. oz.	6
LEMON-PEPPER SEASONING (French's)	1 tsp.	800
LENTIL, whole, dry	1 cup	57
LETTUCE:		
Bibb or Boston	4″ head	15
Cos or Romaine, shredded or broken into pieces	½ cup	2
Grand Rapids, Salad Bowl or Simpson	2 large leaves	4
Iceberg, New York or Great Lakes	¼ of 4¾″ head	10
LIFE, cereal (Quaker):		
Regular	⅔ cup	163
Cinnamon	⅔ cup	149
LIL' ANGELS (Hostess)	1-oz. piece	92
LIME, peeled	2″ dia.	1
***LIMEADE,** frozen (Minute Maid)	6 fl. oz.	<1
LIME JUICE, *ReaLime*	1 T.	<5
LINGUINI WITH CLAM SAUCE, frozen (Stouffer's)	10½ oz.	1010
LIVER:		
Beef:		
Fried	6½″ × 2⅜″ × ⅜″ slice	156
Cooked (Swift)	3.2-oz. serving	70
Calf, fried	6½″ × 2⅜″ × ⅜″ slice	100
Chicken, simmered	2″ × 2″ × ⅝″ liver	15
LIVERWURST SPREAD (Underwood)	1-oz. serving	238

Food and Description	Measure or Quantity	Sodium (mgs.)
LOBSTER:		
Cooked, meat only	1 cup	304
Canned, meat only	4-oz. serving	238
LOBSTER NEWBURG:		
Homemade	1 cup	572
Frozen (Stouffer's)	6½ oz.	700
LOBSTER SALAD	4-oz. serving	141
LOG CABIN SYRUP (See SYRUP)		
LUCKY CHARMS, cereal (General Mills)	1 cup	185
LUNCHEON MEAT (See also individual listings, e.g., BOLOGNA, HAM, etc.)		
All meat (Oscar Mayer)	1-oz. slice	363
Bar-B-Que loaf (Oscar Mayer) 90% fat free	1-oz. slice	374
Beef honey roll sausage (Oscar Mayer) 90% fat free	.8-oz. slice	300
Ham & cheese (See HAM & CHEESE)		
Ham roll sausage (Oscar Mayer)	.8-oz. slice	270
Ham roll sausage (Oscar Mayer)	1-oz. slice	329
Honey Roll (Oscar Mayer) 95% fat free	1-oz. slice	378
Liver cheese (Oscar Mayer)	1.3-oz. slice	456
Luxury loaf (Oscar Mayer) 95% fat free	1-oz. slice	332
New England brand sliced sausage:		
(Oscar Mayer) 92% fat free	.5-oz. slice	180
(Oscar Mayer) 92% fat free	.8-oz. slice	295
Old fashioned loaf (Oscar Mayer)	1-oz. slice	344
Olive loaf, (Oscar Mayer)	1-oz. slice	406
Peppered loaf, (Oscar Mayer) 93% fat free	1-oz. slice	405
Pickle & pimiento (Oscar Mayer)	1-oz. slice	387
Picnic loaf (Oscar Mayer)	1-oz. slice	325
Spiced (Hormel)	1-oz. serving	375

M

MACARONI:
  Cooked

8-10 minutes, firm	1 cup	1
14-20 minutes, tender	1 cup	1

  Canned (Franco-American):

Beefy-Mac	7½-oz. can	900
PizzOs	7½-oz. can	1110

  Frozen:
    (Banquet) & beef:

Regular	12-oz. dinner	2254
Buffet Supper	2-lb. pkg.	5345
(Stouffer's) & beef with tomatoes	5¾ oz.	810
(Swanson) *TV Brand*, & beef	12-oz. dinner	925

MACARONI & CHEESE:

Canned (Franco-American) regular or elbow	7⅜-oz. serving	960

  Frozen:
    (Banquet):

Buffet Supper	2-lb. pkg.	4736
Dinner	12-oz. dinner	1768
(Green Giant) *Boil 'N Bag*	9-oz. entree	1046
(Morton)	8-oz. casserole	909
(Stouffer's)	6 oz.	780

    (Swanson):

Regular	12-oz. entree	1815
TV Brand	12¼-oz. dinner	970
(Van de Kamp's)	10-oz. pkg.	590
*Mix (Prince)	¾ cup	574

MACARONI & CHEESE PIE,

frozen (Swanson)	7-oz. pie	880

MAI TAI COCKTAIL:

Canned (National Distillers) *Duet* 12½% alcohol	8-fl.-oz. can	Tr.

  Mix:

Dry (Bar-Tender's)	1 serving	106

Food and Description	Measure or Quantity	Sodium (mgs.)
MALTED MILK MIX (Carnation):		
Chocolate	3 heaping tsps.	47
Natural	3 heaping tsps.	98
MALT LIQUOR, *Champale*, regular	12 fl. oz.	64
MALT-O-MEAL, cereal	1 T	<1
MANDARIN ORANGE (See TANGERINE)		
MANGO, fresh	1 med. mango	9
MANGO NECTAR (Libby's)	6 fl. oz.	5
MAPLE SYRUP (See SYRUP, Maple)		
MARGARINE:		
Salted:		
(Fleischmann's)	1 T.	111
(Imperial):		
Soft	1 T.	96
Stick	1 T.	112
(Mazola)	1 T.	116
Unsalted (Mazola)	1 T.	<1
MARGARINE, IMITATION OR DIETETIC:		
(Fleischmann's)	1 T.	111
(Mazola)	1·T.	130
MARGARINE, WHIPPED		
(Imperial)	1 T.	62
MARINADE MIX:		
Chicken (Adolph's)	1-oz. packet	4105
Meat:		
(Durkee)	1-oz. pkg.	4104
(French's)	1-oz. pkg.	4320
MARJORAM (French's)	1 tsp.	1
MARMALADE:		
Sweetened (Smucker's)	1 T.	8
Dietetic (Featherweight)	1 T.	45
MARSHMALLOW FLUFF	1 heaping tsp.	5
MARSHMALLOW KRISPIES, cereal (Kellogg's)	1¼ cups	285
MASA HARINA (Quaker)	⅓ cup	2
MASA TRIGO (Quaker)	⅓ cup	294
MATZO (Horowitz Margareten) regular	1 matzo	<1
MAYONNAISE:		
Real, *Hellmann's* (Best Foods)	1 T.	80
Imitation or dietetic:		
(Diet Delight) *Mayo-Lite*	1 T.	75
(Featherweight) *Soyamaise*	1 T.	3

Food and Description	Measure or Quantity	Sodium (mgs.)
MAYPO, cereal:		
30-second	¼ cup	4
Vermont-style	¼ cup	7
McDONALD'S:		
Big Mac	1 hamburger	1010
Biscuit:		
Ham	1 piece	1949
Sausage	1 piece	1380
Cheeseburger	1 hamburger	767
Chicken McNuggets	1 serving	525
Cookies:		
Chocolate Chip	1 package	313
McDonaldland	1 package	358
Egg McMuffin	1 serving	885
Egg, Scrambled	1 serving	205
English Muffin, with butter	1 muffin	318
Filet-O-Fish	1 sandwich	781
Grapefruit Juice	6 fl. oz.	2
Hamburger	1 hamburger	520
Hot cakes with butter & syrup	1 serving	1070
McChicken Sandwich	1 sandwich	990
McFeast	1 serving	678
McRib	1 sandwich	972
Orange Juice	6 fl. oz.	2
Pie:		
Apple	1 pie	398
Cherry	1 pie	427
Potato:		
Fried	1 regular order	109
Hash browns	1 order	325
Quarter Pounder	1 hamburger	735
Quarter Pounder with cheese	1 hamburger	1236
Sausage, pork	1 serving	615
Shake:		
Chocolate	1 serving	300
Strawberry	1 serving	207
Vanilla	1 serving	201
Sundae:		
Caramel	1 sundae	195
Hot Fudge	1 sundae	175
Strawberry	1 sundae	96
MEATBALL DINNER or ENTREE,		
frozen:		
(Green Giant)	9.9-oz. entree	295
(Swanson) *TV Brand*	9¼-oz. entree	1110

Food and Description	Measure or Quantity	Sodium (mgs.)
MEATBALL SANDWICH, frozen		
(Stouffer's)	7¾ oz.	1626
MEATBALL SEASONING MIX:		
*(Durkee) Italian style	1 cup	1019
(French's)	1½-oz. pkg.	3300
MEATBALL STEW, canned,		
(Libby's)	12-oz. serving	1083
MEAT LOAF DINNER, frozen:		
(Banquet):		
Regular	11-oz. dinner	1991
Man-Pleaser	19-oz. dinner	3649
(Swanson):		
TV Brand	10¾-oz. dinner	1130
TV Brand, with tomato sauce		
and whipped potatoes	9-oz. entree	980
MEAT LOAF SEASONING MIX:		
(Contadina)	3¾-oz. pkg.	4301
(French's)	1½-oz. pkg.	4920
MEAT, POTTED (Libby's)	1-oz. serving	297
MEAT SEASONING, dietetic		
(Featherweight)	¼ tsp.	<1
MEAT TENDERIZER:		
(Adolph's)	1 tsp.	1849
(French's) regular	1 tsp.	1760
MELBA TOAST, salted (Old		
London):		
Garlic, onion or white rounds	1 piece	22
Pumpernickel, rye, wheat or white	1 piece	39
Sesame, flat	1 piece	<1
MELON BALL, in syrup, frozen	½ cup	10
MEXICAN DINNER, frozen:		
(Banquet) combination	12-oz. dinner	2346
(Swanson) *TV Brand*	16-oz. dinner	1865
(Van de Kamp's) combination	11-oz. dinner	1504
MILK, CONDENSED	1 T.	21
***MILK, DRY,** non-fat, instant:		
(Alba)	8 fl. oz.	120
(Carnation)	8 fl. oz.	125
Sanalac	8 fl. oz.	100
MILK, EVAPORATED:		
Regular:		
(Carnation)	4 fl. oz.	33
(Pet)	1 fl. oz.	35
Low fat (Carnation)	1 fl. oz.	34
Skimmed (Carnation)	1 fl. oz.	35

Food and Description	Measure or Quantity	Sodium (mgs.)
MILK, FRESH:		
Buttermilk (Friendship) no salt added	8 fl. oz.	140
Chocolate	8 fl. oz.	118
Skim	1 cup	127
Whole	1 cup	122
MILK, GOAT, whole	1 cup	83
MILK, HUMAN	1 oz.	5
MILNOT, dairy vegetable blend	1 fl. oz.	35
MINERAL WATER (Schwepper)	6 fl. oz.	3
MINI-WHEATS, cereal	1 biscuit	1
MINT LEAVES	½ oz.	Tr.
MOLASSES:		
Blackstrap	1 T.	18
Light	1 T.	3
Medium	1 T.	7
Unsulphured (Grandma's)	1 T.	8
MOST, cereal (Kellogg's)	½ cup	145
MUFFIN:		
Blueberry:		
(Hostess)	1¾-oz. piece	149
(Pepperidge Farm)	1.9-oz. piece	250
Bran (Arnold) *Bran'nola*	2.3-oz. muffin	260
Corn:		
(Pepperidge Farm)	1.9-oz. muffin	260
(Thomas')	2-oz. muffin	330
English:		
(Arnold) extra crisp	2.3-oz. muffin	310
(Pepperidge Farm):		
Plain	2-oz. muffin	365
Cinnamon apple	2-oz. muffin	350
Wheat	2-oz. muffin	340
(Thomas') regular or frozen	2-oz. muffin	207
(Wonder)	2-oz. muffin	284
Orange-cranberry (Pepperidge Farm)	2.1-oz. muffin	200
Plain	1.4-oz. muffin	176
Raisin (Arnold)	2.5-oz. muffin	350
Sourdough (Wonder)	2-oz. muffin	128
MUFFIN MIX:		
Blueberry:		
*(Betty Crocker) wild	1 muffin	150
Bran (Duncan Hines)	1/12 of pkg.	161
Cherry (Betty Crocker)	1/12 of pkg.	120
Corn:		
*(Betty Crocker)	1 muffin	315

Food and Description	Measure or Quantity	Sodium (mgs.)
*(Flako)	1 muffin	370
MUSCATEL WINE (Gold Seal) 19% alcohol	3 fl. oz.	3
MUSHROOM:		
Raw, whole	½ lb.	33
Raw, trimmed, sliced	½ cup	5
Canned, solids & liq.		
(Green Giant)	2-oz. serving	258
(Shady Oaks)	4-oz. can	452
Frozen (Green Giant) whole, in butter sauce	3-oz. serving	181
MUSHROOM, CHINESE, dried	1 oz.	11
MUSHROOM SOUP (See SOUP, Mushroom)		
MUSSEL, meat only	1 lb. (weighed in shell)	380
MUSTARD:		
Powder (French's)	1 tsp.	<1
Prepared:		
Brown (French's; Gulden's; *Grey Poupon*)	1 tsp.	48
Dijon, *Grey Poupon*	1 tsp.	149
Horseradish (French's)	1 tsp.	88
Medford (French's)	1 tsp.	80
Mr. Mustard	1 tsp.	90
Unsalted (Featherweight)	1 tsp.	1
Yellow (French's)	1 tsp.	60
MUSTARD GREENS:		
Canned (Sunshine) solids & liq.	½ cup	371
Frozen:		
(Birds Eye)	⅓ of pkg.	27
(McKenzie)	⅓ of pkg.	20
(Southland)	⅕ of 16-oz. pkg.	20

N

NATURAL CEREAL (Quaker):		
100%	¼ cup	11
100% with apple & cinnamon	¼ cup	15
100% with raisins & dates	¼ cup	11

Food and Description	Measure or Quantity	Sodium (mgs.)
NATURE SNACKS (Sun-Maid):		
Carob Crunch	1 oz.	13
Raisin Crunch	1 oz.	41
Rocky Road	1 oz.	4
Tahitian Treat	1 oz.	7
Yogurt Crunch	1 oz.	28
NECTARINE, flesh only	4 oz.	7
NOODLE:		
Dry	1 oz.	1
Cooked, 1½″ strips	1 cup	1
NOODLES & BEEF, frozen		
(Banquet) *Buffet Supper*	2-lb. pkg.	5581
NOODLE & CHICKEN, frozen		
(Swanson) *TV Brand*	10¼-oz. dinner	805
NOODLE, CHOW MEIN (La Choy)	½ cup	206
*NOODLE MIX *(Betty Crocker):		
Fettucini Alfredo	¼ of pkg.	490
Romanoff	¼ of pkg.	705
Stroganoff	¼ of pkg.	605
*NOODLE, RAMEN (La Choy)		
canned:		
Beef	½ of 3-oz. can	1040
Chicken	½ of 3-oz. can	1159
Oriental	½ of 3-oz. can	742
NOODLE, RICE (La Choy)	1 oz.	358
NOODLES ROMANOFF, frozen		
(Stouffer's)	4 oz.	675
NUT, MIXED:		
Dry roasted:		
(Flavor House)	1 oz.	81
(Planters)	1 oz.	222
Oil roasted (Planters)	1 oz.	219
NUTMEG (French's)	1 tsp.	<1
*NUT*Os* (General Mills)	1 T.	55
NUTRI-GRAIN, cereal (Kellogg's):		
Corn	½ cup	185
Wheat	⅔ cup	195

Food and Description	Measure or Quantity	Sodium (mgs.)

O

Food and Description	Measure or Quantity	Sodium (mgs.)
OAT FLAKES, cereal (Post)	⅔ cup	254
OATMEAL:		
Dry:		
Regular:		
(Elam's) Scotch Style	1 oz.	3
(H-O) old fashioned	1 T.	<1
(Quaker) old fashioned	⅓ cup	1
Instant:		
(H-O):		
Regular, boxed	1 T.	<1
Regular, packets	1-oz. packet	230
With bran & spice	1½-oz. packet	297
With cinnamon & spice	1⅝-oz. packet	306
With maple & brown sugar		
flavor	1½-oz. packet	286
Sweet & mellow	1.4-oz. packet	270
(Quaker):		
Regular	1-oz. packet	281
Apple & cinnamon	1¼-oz. packet	181
Bran & raisin	1½-oz. packet	240
Maple & brown sugar	1½-oz. packet	228
Raisins & spice	1½-oz. packet	217
(3-Minute Brand) *Stir 'N Eat:*		
Dutch apple brown sugar	1⅛-oz. packet	205
Natural flavor	1-oz. packet	230
Quick:		
(Harvest Brand)	⅓ cup	3
(H-O)	½ cup	<1
(Quaker) old fashioned	⅓ cup	1
(Ralston Purina)	⅓ cup	3
(3-Minute Brand)	⅓ cup	3
*Cooked, regular	1 cup	523
OIL, SALAD or COOKING	Any quantity	0
OKRA, frozen:		
(Birds Eye) whole	⅓ of pkg.	2
(Green Giant) gumbo	⅓ of pkg.	334

Food and Description	Measure or Quantity	Sodium (mgs.)
(McKenzie) cut	⅓ of pkg.	3
(Southland) cut	⅕ of 16-oz. pkg.	3
OLD FASHIONED COCKTAIL, mix, dry (Bar-Tender's)	1 serving	Tr.
OLIVE:		
Green	4 med. or 3 extra large or 2 giant	384
Ripe, Mission	3 small or 2 large	75
OMELET, frozen (Swanson) *TV Brand,* Spanish style	7¾-oz. entree	905
ONION:		
Raw	2½" onion	10
Boiled, pearl onion	½ cup	6
Canned (Durkee) *O & C:*		
Boiled	¼ of 16-oz. jar	8
Creamed	¼ of 15½-oz. jar	11,059
Dehydrated (Gilroy) flakes	1 tsp.	1
Frozen:		
(Birds Eye):		
Chopped	1 oz.	2
Creamed	⅓ of pkg.	333
Whole	⅓ of pkg.	11
(Green Giant) cheese sauce	⅓ of pkg.	268
(Mrs. Paul's) french-fried rings	½ of 5-oz. pkg.	625
(Southland) chopped	⅕ of 10-oz. pkg.	17
ONION BOUILLON:		
(Herb-Ox)	1 cube	560
MBT	1 packet	795
ONION, GREEN	1 small onion	<1
ONION SALAD SEASONING (French's) instant	1 T.	2
ONION SOUP, canned (See SOUP, Onion)		
ON*YOS (General Mills)	1 T.	45
ORANGE:		
Peeled	½ cup	1
Sections	4 oz.	1
ORANGE DRINK:		
Canned:		
Capri Sun	6¾-oz. can	2
(Hi-C)	8 fl. oz.	77
*Mix (Hi-C)	8 fl. oz.	1
ORANGE EXTRACT (Virginia Dare)	1 tsp.	0

Food and Description	Measure or Quantity	Sodium (mgs.)
ORANGE-GRAPEFRUIT JUICE:		
Canned (Del Monte)	6 fl. oz.	2
*Frozen (Minute Maid) unsweetened	6 fl. oz.	<1
ORANGE JUICE:		
Canned:		
(Del Monte) sweetened	6 fl. oz.	2
(Libby's) sweetened	6 fl. oz.	5
(Texsun) sweetened	6 fl. oz.	2
Chilled (Minute Maid)	6 fl. oz.	1
*Frozen:		
(Minute Maid) unsweetened	6 fl. oz.	1
(Snow Crop)	6 fl. oz.	1
ORANGE-PINEAPPLE JUICE,		
canned (Texsun)	6 fl. oz.	2
ORANGE PLUS (Birds Eye)	6 fl. oz.	9
ORANGE SPREAD, dietetic (Estee)	1 tsp.	<1
OVALTINE:		
Chocolate	¾ oz.	146
Malt	¾ oz.	92
OVEN FRY (General Foods):		
Crispy crumb for pork	4.2-oz. envelope	2780
Extra crispy for chicken	4.2-oz. envelope	3801
Traditional pork	5.3-oz. envelope	4943
OYSTER:		
Raw, Eastern	19-31 small or 13-19 med.	175
Fried	4 oz.	234
OYSTER STEW, home recipe	½ cup	243

P

PAC-MAN CEREAL (General Mills)	1 cup	195
PANCAKE BATTER, frozen		
(Aunt Jemima):		
Plain	4″ pancake	286
Blueberry	4″ pancake	233
Buttermilk	4″ pancake	244
PANCAKE & SAUSAGE, frozen		
(Swanson)	6-oz. entree	985

Food and Description	Measure or Quantity	Sodium (mgs.)
*PANCAKE & WAFFLE MIX:		
Plain:		
(Aunt Jemima):		
Complete	4″ pancake	290
Original	4″ pancake	183
(Log Cabin):		
Complete	4″ pancake	203
Original	4″ pancake	180
(Pillsbury) *Hungry Jack:*		
Complete, bulk or packets	4″ pancake	235
Extra Lights	4″ pancake	165
Panshakes	4″ pancake	293
Blueberry (Pillsbury) *Hungry Jack*	4″ pancake	272
Buckwheat (Aunt Jemima)	4″ pancake	173
Buttermilk:		
(Aunt Jemima):		
Regular	4″ pancake	330
Complete	4″ pancake	290
(Betty Crocker):		
Regular	4″ pancake	270
Complete	4″ pancake	193
(Pillsbury) *Hungry Jack,* complete	4″ pancake	235
Whole wheat (Aunt Jemima)	4″ pancake	242
Dietetic (Featherweight)	4″ pancake	23
PANCAKE & WAFFLE SYRUP (See SYRUP, Pancake & Waffle)		
PAPAYA, fresh:		
Cubed	½ cup	2
Juice	4 oz.	35
PAPRIKA (French's)	1 tsp.	<1
PARSLEY:		
Fresh, chopped	1 T.	2
Dried (French's)	1 tsp.	6
PASTINAS, egg	1 oz.	1
PASTRY SHEET, PUFF, frozen (Pepperidge Farm)	4.3-oz. sheet	580
PASTRY SHELL, frozen (Pepperidge Farm)	1 patty shell	180
PEA, green:		
Boiled	½ cup	1
Canned, regular pack, solids & liq.:		
(Del Monte):		
Early	½ cup	331
Seasoned	½ cup	302

Food and Description	Measure or Quantity	Sodium (mgs.)
(Green Giant):		
Early, with onions	½ cup	534
Sweet	½ cup	339
(Libby's) sweet	½ cup	337
(Stokely-Van Camp) early	½ cup	375
Canned, dietetic pack, solids & liq.:		
(Diet Delight)	½ cup	5
(Featherweight) sweet	½ cup	<10
(S&W) *Nutradiet*, sweet	½ cup	<10
Frozen:		
(Birds Eye):		
Regular	3.3 oz.	95
In cream sauce	2.7 oz.	446
With sliced mushrooms	3.3 oz.	214
(Green Giant):		
Creamed	3.3 oz.	267
Early & sweet in butter sauce	3.3 oz.	442
Sweet, *Harvest Fresh*	4-oz. serving	299
Sweet, polybag	3 oz.	28
(McKenzie):		
Regular	3.3 oz.	91
Tiny	3.3 oz.	127
PEA & CARROT:		
Canned, regular pack, solids & liq.:		
(Del Monte)	½ cup	313
(Libby's)	½ cup	315
Canned, dietetic pack, solids & liq.:		
(Diet Delight)	½ cup	5
(S&W) *Nutradiet*	½ cup	<10
Frozen (Birds Eye)	⅓ of pkg.	69
PEA, CROWDER, frozen (Birds Eye)	⅕ of 16-oz. pkg.	6
PEA & ONION, frozen (Birds Eye)		
PEA SOUP, GREEN (See SOUP, Pea)		
PEACH:		
Fresh, with thin skin	2″ peach	1
Fresh, slices	½ cup	1
Canned, regular pack, solids & liq.:		
(Del Monte):		
Cling	½ cup	3
Spiced	7¼ oz.	8
(Libby's):		
Halves, heavy syrup	½ cup	9
Sliced, heavy syrup	½ cup	10

Food and Description	Measure or Quantity	Sodium (mgs.)
Canned, dietetic pack, solids & liq.:		
(Del Monte) *Lite*, Cling	½ cup	6
(Diet Delight) cling, syrup pack	½ cup	10
(Featherweight) cling or		
Freestone, juice or water pack	½ cup	<10
(Libby's) Lite	½ cup	10
Frozen (Birds Eye) sliced	5 oz.	9
PEACH BUTTER (Smucker's)	1 T.	2
PEACH DRINK (Hi-C):		
Canned	6 fl. oz.	<1
*Mix	6 fl. oz.	17
PEACH NECTAR (Libby's)	6 fl. oz.	5
PEACH PRESERVE OR JAM:		
Sweetened (Smucker's)	1 T.	4
Dietetic (Featherweight)	1 T.	45
PEANUT:		
Dry roasted:		
(Fisher) salted	1 oz.	101
(Planters) salted	1 oz.	222
Oil roasted (Planters), salted	1 oz. (jar)	219
PEANUT BUTTER:		
Regular:		
(Elam's) Natural with defatted		
wheat germ	1 T.	4
(Jif) creamy	1 T.	89
(Peter Pan):		
Crunchy	1 T.	59
Smooth	1 T.	92
(Planters) crunchy or smooth	1 T.	94
(Skippy):		
Creamy	1 T.	80
Creamy, old fashioned or super		
chunk	1 T.	75
Dietetic, low sodium:		
(Featherweight)	1 T.	<5
(Peter Pan)	1 T.	Tr.
(S&W) *Nutradiet*	1 T.	<10
PEANUT BUTTER BAKING CHIPS		
(Reese's)	3 T. (1 oz.)	61
PEAR:		
Whole	3″ × 2½″ pear	3
Canned, regular pack, solids & liq.:		
(Del Monte)	½ cup	6
(Libby's)	½ cup	6

Food and Description	Measure or Quantity	Sodium (mgs.)
Canned, dietetic pack, solids & liq.:		
(Del Monte) *Lite*	½ cup	2
(Featherweight) Bartlett, juice or water pack	½ cup	5
(Libby's) water pack	½ cup	10
Dried (Sun-Maid)	½ cup	7
PEAR NECTAR (Libby's)	6 fl. oz.	5
PEBBLES, cereal:		
Cocoa	⅞ cup	136
Fruity	⅞ cup	158
PECAN:		
Halves	6–7 pieces	Tr.
Roasted, dry:		
(Fisher) salted	1 oz.	110
(Planters) salted	1 oz.	222
PECTIN, FRUIT:		
Certo	6 oz.	5
Sure-Jell	1¾ oz.	12
PEP, cereal (Kellogg's)	¾ cup	200
PEPPER:		
Black (French's)	1 tsp.	<1
Seasoned (French's)	1 tsp.	5
PEPPER, CHILI, canned:		
(*Del Monte*):		
Green, whole	½ cup	819
Jalapeno or chili, whole	½ cup	1653
(Ortega):		
Diced, strips or whole	1 oz.	20
Jalapeno, diced or whole	1 oz.	6
PEPPERONI:		
(Hormel) sliced	1-oz. serving	508
(Swift)	1-oz. serving	579
PEPPER STEAK, frozen (Stouffer's)	5¼-oz. serving	750
PEPPER STUFFED:		
Home recipe	2¾″ × 2½″ pepper with 1⅛ cups stuffing	581
Frozen:		
(Green Giant) green, baked	7 oz.	851
(Stouffer's)	7¾ oz.	960
(Weight Watchers) with veal stuffing	11¾ oz.	1004
PEPPER, SWEET:		
Raw:		
Green:		
Whole	1 lb.	48

Food and Description	Measure or Quantity	Sodium (mgs.)
Without stem & seeds	1 med. pepper (2.6 oz.)	8
Frozen: (McKenzie) green	1 oz.	1
PERCH, OCEAN:		
Atlantic, raw:		
Whole	1 lb.	111
Meat only	4 oz.	71
Pacific, raw, whole	1 lb.	77
Frozen:		
(Banquet)	8¾-oz. dinner	1416
(Mrs. Paul's) fillet, breaded & fried	2-oz. piece	400
(Weight Watchers)	6½-oz. meal	480
PERSIMMON:		
Japanese or Kaki, fresh:		
With seeds	4.4-oz. piece	6
Seedless	4.4-oz. piece	6
Native, fresh, flesh only	4 oz.	1
PICKLE:		
Cucumber, fresh or bread & butter:		
(Fanning's)	1.2 oz.	189
(Featherweight)	1 oz.	3
Dill:		
(USDA)	4″ × 1¾″ piece (4.8 oz.)	1928
(Featherweight) whole, low sodium	1 oz.	<5
(Smucker's):		
Candied sticks	4″ stick	182
Hamburger sliced	1 slice	141
Kosher dill:		
(Claussen) halves or whole	2 oz.	599
(Featherweight) low sodium	1 oz.	<5
(Smucker's) whole	2½″ piece	642
Sweet:		
(Aunt Jane's)	1½ oz. piece	420
(Smucker's) whole	2½″ long pickle	119
Sweet & sour (Claussen) slices	1 slice	25
PIE:		
Regular:		
Apple:		
Home recipe, two-crust	⅙ of 9″ pie	476
(Hostess)	4½-oz. pie	563
Banana, home recipe, cream or custard	⅙ of 9″ pie	295
Berry (Hostess)	4½-oz. pie	415

Food and Description	Measure or Quantity	Sodium (mgs.)
Blackberry, home recipe, two-crust	⅙ of 9" pie	423
Blueberry:		
Home recipe, two-crust	⅙ of 9" pie	423
(Hostess)	4½-oz. pie	415
Boston cream, home recipe	1/12 of 8" pie	128
Butterscotch, home recipe, one-crust	⅙ of 9" pie	325
Cherry:		
Home recipe, two-crust	⅙ of 9" pie	480
(Hostess)	4½-oz. pie	537
Chocolate chiffon, home recipe	⅙ of 9" pie	353
Chocolate meringue, home recipe	⅙ of 9" pie	358
Coconut custard, home recipe	⅙ of 9" pie	375
Lemon (Hostess)	4½-oz. pie	422
Mince, home recipe, two-crust	⅙ of 9" pie	708
Peach (Hostess)	4½-oz. pie	447
Pecan (Frito-Lay)	3-oz. serving	453
Pumpkin, home recipe, one-crust	⅙ of 9" pie	325
Raisin, home recipe, two-crust	⅙ of 9" pie	450
Rhubarb, home recipe, two-crust	⅙ of 9" pie	427
Strawberry (Hostess)	4½-oz. pie	396
Frozen:		
Apple:		
(Banquet)	⅕ of 20-oz. pie	358
(Morton) regular	⅙ of 24-oz. pie	239
(Sara Lee):		
Regular	⅙ of 31-oz. pie	280
Dutch	⅙ of 30-oz. pie	282
Banana cream:		
(Banquet)	⅙ of 14-oz. pie	77
(Morton):		
Regular	⅙ of 16-oz. pie	123
Blueberry:		
(Banquet)	⅙ of 20-oz. pie	263
(Morton) regular	⅙ of 24-oz. pie	250
(Sara Lee)	⅙ of 31-oz. pie	220
Cherry:		
(Banquet)	⅙ of 20-oz. pie	294
(Morton) regular	⅙ of 24-oz. pie	250
(Sara Lee)	⅙ of 31-oz. pie	233
Cherry:		
(Banquet)	⅙ of 20-oz. pie	294
(Morton) regular	⅙ of 24-oz. pie	250
(Sara Lee)	⅙ of 31-oz. pie	233

Food and Description	*Measure or Quantity*	*Sodium (mgs.)*
Chocolate cream:		
(Banquet)	1/6 of 14-oz. pie	64
(Morton) regular	1/6 of 16-oz. pie	129
Coconut cream:		
(Banquet)	1/6 of 14-oz. pie	65
(Morton) regular	1/6 of 16-oz. pie	122
Coconut custard:		
(Banquet)	1/6 of 20-oz. pie	297
Custard (Banquet)	1/5 of 20-oz. pie	347
Lemon cream:		
(Banquet)	1/6 of 14-oz. pie	66
(Morton) regular	1/6 of 16-oz. pie	121
Mince:		
(Banquet)	1/6 of 20-oz. pie	459
(Morton)	1/6 of 24-oz. pie	352
Peach:		
(Banquet)	1/5 of 20-oz. pie	329
(Morton)	1/6 of 24-oz. pie	263
(Sara Lee)	1/6 of 31-oz. pie	253
Pumpkin:		
(Banquet)	1/6 of 20-oz. pie	222
(Morton)	1/6 of 24-oz. pie	309
(Sara Lee)	1/8 of 45-oz. pie	403
Strawberry cream:		
(Banquet)	1/6 of 14-oz. pie	83
(Morton)	1/6 of 16-oz. pie	122
PIECRUST:		
Home recipe, 9″ pie	1 crust	1100
Frozen (Banquet) 9″ pie shell:		
Regular	1 crust	960
Deep dish	1 crust	936
***PIECRUST MIX:**		
(Betty Crocker) regular or stick:		
Regular	1/16 pkg.	140
Stick	1/8 stick	140
(Flako)	1/6 of 9″ pie shell	314
(Pillsbury) mix or stick	1/6 of 2-crust shell	425
PIE FILLING (See also PUDDING or PIE FILLING):		
Apple (Comstock)	1/6 of 21-oz. can	150
Apple rings or slices (See APPLE, canned)		
Apricot (Comstock)	1/6 of 21-oz. can	250
Banana cream (Comstock)	1/6 of 21-oz. can	700
Blueberry (Comstock)	1/6 of 21-oz. can	350
Cherry (Comstock)	1/6 of 21-oz. can	400

Food and Description	Measure or Quantity	Sodium (mgs.)
Chocolate (Comstock)	⅙ of 21-oz. can	600
Coconut cream (Comstock)	⅙ of 21-oz. can	650
Coconut custard, home recipe, made with egg yolk & milk	5 oz. (inc. crust)	334
Lemon (Comstock)	⅙ of 21-oz. can	300
Peach (Comstock)	⅙ of 21-oz. can	250
Pineapple (Comstock)	⅙ of 21-oz. can	150
Pumpkin (Libby's) (See also PUMPKIN, canned)	1 cup	420
Raisin (Comstock)	⅙ of 21-oz. can	200
Strawberry (Comstock)	⅙ of 21-oz. can	200
*PIE MIX (Betty Crocker) Boston cream	⅛ of pie	405
PIEROGIES, frozen (Mrs. Paul's):		
Cabbage	5-oz. serving	650
Potato & cheese	5-oz. serving	550
Sauerkraut, Polish-style	5-oz. serving	400
PIMIENTO, canned:		
(Ortega)	¼ cup	18
(Sunshine) diced or sliced	1 T.	3
PINEAPPLE:		
Fresh, slices	½ cup	<1
Canned, regular pack, solids & liq.:		
(Del Monte) slices, medium	½ cup	2
(Dole):		
Chunk, crushed or sliced, juice pack	½ cup	1
Chunk, crushed or sliced, heavy syrup	½ cup	2
Canned, unsweetened or dietetic, solids & liq.:		
(Del Monte):		
Chunks, juice pack	½ cup	1
Crushed, juice pack	½ cup	1
Slices, juice pack	½ cup	1
(Diet Delight) juice pack	½ cup	5
(Featherweight) juice or water pack	½ cup	<10
(Libby's)	½ cup	10
PINEAPPLE & GRAPEFRUIT JUICE DRINK, canned:		
(Del Monte) regular or pink	6 fl. oz.	43
(Dole) pink	6 fl. oz.	Tr.
(Texson)	6 fl. oz.	2

Food and Description	Measure or Quantity	Sodium (mgs.)
PINEAPPLE JUICE:		
Canned:		
(Del Monte) with vitamin C	6 fl. oz.	4
(Dole)	6 fl. oz.	2
(Texson)	6 fl. oz.	2
*Frozen (Minute Maid)	6 fl. oz.	2
PINEAPPLE-ORANGE DRINK,		
canned (Hi-C)	6 fl. oz.	<1
PINEAPPLE-ORANGE JUICE:		
Canned (Del Monte)	6 fl. oz.	6
*Frozen (Minute Maid)	6 fl. oz.	2
PINEAPPLE PRESERVE OR JAM,		
sweetened (Smucker's)	1 T.	1
PISTACHIO NUT (Fisher) in shell,		
salted	1 oz.	50
PIZZA PIE:		
Regular, non-frozen:		
Home recipe with cheese topping	⅛ of 14″ pie	527
(Pizza Hut):		
Cheese	½ of 10″ pie	1431
Pepperoni	½ of 10″ pie	1638
Pork	½ of 10″ pie	1719
Frozen:		
Cheese:		
(Celeste)	½ of 7-oz. pie	655
(Celeste)	¼ of 19-oz. pie	803
(Stouffer's) French bread	½ of 10¼-oz. pkg.	850
Totino's	½ of pie	1130
(Weight Watchers)	6-oz. pie	914
Combination:		
(Celeste) Chicago style	¼ of 24-oz. pie	1156
(La Pizzeria)	½ of 13½-oz. pie	959
(Van de Kamp's) thick crust	¼ of 23.4-oz. pie	614
(Weight Watchers) deluxe	7¼-oz. pie	690
Deluxe:		
(Celeste)	½ of 9-oz. pie	794
(Celeste)	¼ of 23½-oz. pie	1049
(Stouffer's) French bread	½ of 12⅜-oz. pkg.	1150
Hamburger (Stouffer's) French		
bread	½ of 12¼-oz. pkg.	1100
Mexican Style (Van de Kamp's)	½ of 11-oz. pie	569
Pepperoni:		
(Celeste)	½ of 7¼-oz. pie	888
(Celeste)	¼ of 20-oz. pie	1082
(Stouffer's) French bread	½ of 11¼-oz. pkg.	1190
Totino's	½ of pie	1350

Food and Description	Measure or Quantity	Sodium (mgs.)
(Van de Kamp's) thick crust	¼ of 22-oz. pie	651
Sausage:		
(Celeste)	½ of 8-oz. pie	764
(Celeste)	¼ of 22-oz. pie	1227
(Stouffer's) French bread	½ of 12-oz. pkg.	1320
Totino's	½ of pie	1260
Totino's, deep crust	⅙ of pie	765
(Weight Watchers)	6¾-oz. pie	876
Sausage & mushroom:		
(Celeste)	½ of 9-oz. pie	788
(Celeste)	¼ of 24-oz. pie	1195
(Stouffer's) French bread	½ of 12½-oz. pkg.	1220
Sicilian style (Celeste) deluxe	¼ of 26-oz. pie	1190
Vegetable (Weight Watchers)	7¼-oz. pie	727
*PIZZA PIE MIX (Ragu) *Pizza Quick*	⅛ of 12″ pie	370
PIZZA SAUCE (Contadina):		
Regular	½ cup	700
with cheese	½ cup	750
PIZZA SEASONING SPICE (French's)	1 tsp.	390
PLUM:		
Fresh, Japanese & hybrid	2″ plum	<1
Fresh, prune-type, halves	½ cup	<1
Canned, regular pack (Stokely-Van Camp)	½ cup	28
Canned, purple, unsweetened or dietetic, solids & liq.:		
(Diet Delight) juice pack	½ cup	5
(Featherweight) juice or water pack	½ cup	<10
PLUM JELLY (Featherweight)	1 T.	45
PLUM PRESERVE OR JAM, sweetened (Smucker's)	1 T.	3
POLYNESIAN-STYLE DINNER, frozen (Swanson) *TV Brand*	12-oz. dinner	1355
POMEGRANATE, whole	1 lb.	8
PONDEROSA RESTAURANT:		
A-1 sauce	1 tsp.	82
Beef, chopped (patty only):		
Regular	3½ oz.	58
Big	4.8 oz.	81
Double Deluxe	5.9 oz.	99
Junior (*Square Shooter*)	1.6 oz.	27
Steakhouse Deluxe	2.96 oz.	50

Food and Description	Measure or Quantity	Sodium (mgs.)
Beverages:		
Coca-Cola	8 fl. oz.	1
Coffee	6 fl. oz.	26
Dr. Pepper	8 fl. oz.	18
Milk:		
Regular	8 fl. oz.	122
Chocolate	8 fl. oz.	149
Orange drink	8 fl. oz.	12
Root beer	8 fl. oz.	18
Sprite	8 fl. oz.	31
Tab	8 fl. oz.	18
Bun:		
Regular	2.4-oz. bun	334
Hot dog	1 bun	263
Junior	1.4-oz. bun	197
Steakhouse Deluxe	2.4-oz. bun	334
Butter	1 pat (1 tsp.)	49
Catsup	1 T.	143
Chicken strips:		
Adult	2¾ oz.	420
Child	1.4 oz.	210
Cocktail sauce	1½ oz.	143
Filet Mignon	3.8 oz. (edible portion)	82
Filet of Sole, fish only (see also Bun)	3-oz. piece	46
Fish, baked	4.9-oz. serving	363
Gelatin dessert	½ cup	55
Gravy, Au Jus	1 oz.	125
Ham & cheese:		
Bun (See Bun)		
Cheese, Swiss	2 slices (.8 oz.)	310
Ham	2½ oz.	724
Hot dog, child's, meat only (see also Bun)	1.6-oz. hot dog	542
Lemon wedge	1 piece	<1
Lettuce (see Salad Bar)		
Margarine:		
Pat	1 tsp.	49
On potato, as served	½ oz.	138
Mayonnaise	1 T.	84
Mustard	1 T.	189
New York strip steak	6.1 oz. (edible portion)	79
Onion, chopped	1 T. (.4 oz.)	1

85

Food and Description	Measure or Quantity	Sodium (mgs.)
Pickle, dill	3 slices (.7 oz.)	279
Potato:		
Baked	7.2 oz.	6
French fries	3 oz.	5
Prime Rib:		
Regular	4.2 oz. (edible portion)	71
Imperial	8.4 oz. (edible portion)	141
King	6 oz. (edible portion)	101
Pudding:		
Butterscotch	4½ oz.	192
Chocolate	4½ oz.	177
Vanilla	4½ oz.	127
Ribeye	3.2 oz. (edible portion)	271
Ribeye & Shrimp:		
Ribeye	3.2 oz.	271
Shrimp	2.2 oz.	114
Roll, kaiser	2.2-oz. roll	322
Salad bar:		
Beets	1 oz.	56
Broccoli	1 oz.	4
Cabbage, red	1 oz.	7
Carrots	1 oz.	13
Cauliflower	1 oz.	4
Celery	1 oz.	36
Chickpeas (Garbanzos)	1 oz.	7
Cucumber	1 oz.	2
Lettuce	1 oz.	3
Mushrooms	1 oz.	4
Onions, white	1 oz.	3
Pepper, green	1 oz.	4
Radish	1 oz.	5
Tomato	1 oz.	<1
Salad dressing:		
Blue cheese	1 oz.	265
Italian, creamy	1 oz.	419
Low calorie	1 oz.	220
Oil & vinegar	1 oz.	<1
Sweet'n tart	1 oz.	340
Thousand island	1 oz.	170
Shrimp dinner	7 pieces (3½ oz.)	182

Food and Description	Measure or Quantity	Sodium (mgs.)
Sirloin:		
Regular	3.3 oz. (edible portion)	182
Super	6½ oz. (edible portion)	695
Tips	4 oz. (edible portion)	375
Steak sauce	1 oz.	329
Tartar sauce	1½ oz.	300
T-Bone	4.3 oz. (edible portion)	545
Tomato (see also Salad bar):		
Slices	2 slices (.9 oz.)	7
Whole, small	3.5 oz.	3
Topping, whipped	¼ oz.	4
POPCORN		
*Home made, popped:		
(Jiffy Pop)	½ of 5-oz. pkg.	936
(Pillsbury) Microwave Popcorn:		
Regular	1 cup	129
Butter flavor	1 cup	176
Packaged, caramel-coated (Old London):		
Without peanuts	1¾-oz. bag	372
With peanuts	1 cup	258
***POPOVER MIX** (Flako)	1 popover	255
POPPY SEED (French's)	1 tsp.	<1
POP TARTS (See TOASTER CAKE OR PASTRY)		
PORK:		
Fresh:		
Chop:		
Broiled, lean & fat	3-oz. chop (weighed without bone)	55
Broiled, lean only	3-oz. chop (weighed without bone)	55
Loin:		
Roasted, lean & fat	3 oz.	56
Roasted, lean only	3 oz.	56
Spareribs, braised	3 oz.	55
Cured ham, roasted, lean only	3 oz.	791
PORK DINNER (Swanson) *TV Brand*	11¼-oz. dinner	595
PORK RINDS, *Baken-Ets*	1-oz. serving	245
PORK, SWEET & SOUR, frozen (La Choy)	½ of 15-oz. pkg.	1586

Food and Description	Measure or Quantity	Sodium (mgs.)
PORT WINE:		
(Gold Seal)	3 fl. oz.	3
(Great Western)	3 fl. oz.	34
***POSTUM,** instant	6 fl. oz.	3
POTATO:		
Cooked:		
Au gratin	½ cup	433
Baked, peeled	2½″ dia. potato	4
Boiled, peeled	4.2-oz. potato	288
French-fried, no added salt	10 pieces	3
Hash-browned, home recipe	½ cup	281
Mashed, milk & butter added	½ cup	324
Canned:		
(Del Monte) drained	1 cup	812
(Sunshine) whole, solids & liq.	1 cup	753
Frozen:		
(Birds Eye):		
Cottage fries	2.8-oz. serving	14
Crinkle cuts, regular	3-oz. serving	36
French fries, regular	3-oz. serving	23
Hash browns, regular	¼ of 16-oz. pkg.	54
Tasti Puffs	¼ of 10-oz. pkg.	401
Tiny Taters	⅕ of 16-oz. pkg.	282
Triangles	1½-oz. serving	167
(Green Giant):		
Sliced in butter sauce	3.3 oz.	309
& sweet peas in bacon cream sauce	3.3 oz.	335
(McKenzie) whole, white	3.2 oz.	5
(Stouffer's)		
Au gratin	⅓ of pkg.	480
Scalloped	⅓ of pkg.	450
POTATO CHIP:		
(Featherweight) unsalted	1 oz.	6
(Frito-Lay's) natural	1 oz.	265
Lay's, sour cream & onion flavor	1 oz.	407
(Planter's) stackable	1 oz.	222
Pringle's:		
Regular	1 oz.	216
Light	1 oz.	143
Rippled	1 oz.	247
***POTATO MIX:**		
Au gratin:		
(Betty Crocker)	½ cup	605
(French's) *Big Tate*, tangy	½ cup	525

Food and Description	Measure or Quantity	Sodium (mgs.)
Creamed (Betty Crocker)	½ cup	385
Hash browns (Betty Crocker) with onion	½ cup	460
Hickory smoke cheese (Betty Crocker)	½ cup	650
Julienne (Betty Crocker) with mild cheese sauce	½ cup	570
Mashed:		
(American Beauty)	½ cup	340
(Betty Crocker) *Buds*	½ cup	355
(French's) *Big Tate*	½ cup	365
(Pillsbury) *Hungry Jack*, flakes	½ cup	370
Scalloped:		
(Betty Crocker)	½ cup	570
(French's) *Big Tate*	½ cup	520
Sour cream & chive (Betty Crocker)	½ cup	495
*POTATO PANCAKE MIX		
(French's) *Big Tate*	3" pancake	163
POTATO SALAD, home recipe	½ cup	600
POTATO STICK (Durkee) *O & C*	1½-oz. can	383
POTATO, STUFFED, BAKED, frozen (Green Giant) with cheese topping	½ potato	510
POUND CAKE (See CAKE, Pound)		
PRETZEL:		
(Featherweight) unsalted	1 piece	1
(Pepperidge Farm):		
Nuggets	1¼-oz. serving	497
Twists, tiny	1 oz.	366
(Rokeach) *Baldies*, unsalted	1 oz.	30
PRODUCT 19, cereal (Kellogg's)	¾ cup	315
PRUNE:		
Canned:		
(Del Monte):		
Moist-Pak	2 oz.	2
Stewed	4 oz.	1
(Featherweight) water pack	½ cup	<10
(Sunsweet) stewed	½ cup	2
Dried:		
(Del Monte):		
Breakfast, medium, large or pitted	2 oz.	2
Jumbo	2 oz.	1
(Sunsweet) whole	2 oz.	5
PRUNE JUICE:		
(Del Monte)	6 fl. oz.	4

Food and Description	Measure or Quantity	Sodium (mgs.)
(Sunsweet) regular or with pulp	6 fl. oz.	15
PRUNE WHIP, home recipe	½ cup	221
PUDDING OR PIE FILLING:		
Canned, regular pack:		
Banana (Del Monte) *Pudding Cup*	5-oz. container	277
Butterscotch (Del Monte) *Pudding Cup*	5-oz. container	277
Chocolate:		
(Del Monte) *Pudding Cup*	5-oz. container	327
(Hunt's) *Snack Pack*	5-oz. container	146
Rice:		
Home recipe, with raisins	½ cup	94
(Comstock)	½ of 7½-oz. can	450
(Hunt's) *Snack Pack*	5-oz. container	192
(Menner's)	½ of 7½-oz. can	450
Tapioca:		
Home recipe, cream	½ cup	128
(Del Monte) *Pudding Cup*	5-oz. container	253
(Hunt's) *Snack Pack*	5-oz. container	210
Vanilla (Del Monte)	5-oz. container	320
Chilled, *Swiss Miss:*		
Butterscotch, chocolate malt or vanilla	4-oz. container	175
Chocolate	4-oz. container	176
Rice	4-oz. container	296
Tapioca	4-oz. container	170
Frozen (Rich's):		
Banana	3-oz. container	118
Butterscotch	4½-oz. container	192
Chocolate	4½-oz. container	205
Vanilla	4½-oz. container	243
Mix, sweetened, regular & instant:		
Banana:		
*(Jell-O)		
Regular	½ cup	257
Instant	½ cup	437
*(Royal):		
Regular	½ cup	229
Instant	½ cup	243
*Butter Pecan (Jell-O) instant	½ cup	442
Butterscotch:		
*(Jell-O):		
Regular	½ cup	244
Instant	½ cup	474
*(Royal) regular	½ cup	229

Food and Description	Measure or Quantity	Sodium (mgs.)
Chocolate:		
*(Jell-O) regular	½ cup	192
*(Royal):		
Regular	½ cup	143
Instant	½ cup	365
Coconut:		
*(Jell-O) cream, regular	½ cup	216
*(Royal) instant	½ cup	323
Custard (Royal) regular	½ cup	131
*Flan (Royal) regular	½ cup	131
Lemon:		
*(Jell-O) instant	½ cup	387
*(Royal) regular	½ cup	94
*Lime (Royal) Key Lime, regular	½ cup	94
*Pineapple (Jell-O) cream, regular	½ cup	393
*Pistachio (Royal) nut, instant	½ cup	323
*Raspberry (Salada) *Danish Dessert*	½ cup	5
*Rice, *Jell-O Americana*	½ cup	158
Tapioca:		
Jell-O Americana, chocolate or vanilla	½ cup	170
*(Royal) chocolate	½ cup	143
Vanilla:		
*(Jell-O) regular	½ cup	198
*(Jell-O) French, regular	½ cup	436
*(Royal) regular	½ cup	229
*Mix, dietetic:		
Butterscotch:		
(D-Zerta)	½ cup	148
(Featherweight) artificially sweetened	½ cup	70
Chocolate:		
(D-Zerta)	½ cup	82
(Estee)	½ cup	Tr.
(Featherweight) artificially sweetened	½ cup	78
Lemon (Estee)	½ cup	Tr.
Vanilla:		
(D-Zerta)	½ cup	133
(Estee)	½ cup	9
(Featherweight) artificially sweetened	½ cup	70
PUFFED RICE:		
(Malt-O-Meal)	1 cup	1

Food and Description	Measure or Quantity	Sodium (mgs.)
(Quaker)	1 cup	1
PUFFED WHEAT:		
(Malt-O-Meal)	1 cup	1
(Quaker)	1 cup	1
PUMPKIN, canned:		
(Del Monte)	½ cup	6
(Libby's) solid pack	½ cup	10

Q

QUAIL, raw, meat & skin	4 oz.	45
QUIK (Nestlé):		
Chocolate	1 T.	18
Strawberry	1 T.	<5
QUISP, cereal	1⅙ cups	189

R

RADISH	2 small radishes	3
RAISIN, dried:		
(Del Monte)	3 oz.	9
(Sun-Maid)	3 oz.	10
RAISINS, RICE & RYE, cereal		
(Kellogg's)	¾ cup	250
RALSTON, cereal	¼ cup	3
RASPBERRY:		
Fresh:		
Black, trimmed	½ cup	<1
Red, trimmed	½ cup	<1
Frozen (Birds Eye) quick thaw	5-oz. serving	1
RASPBERRY PRESERVE OR JAM, sweetened (Smucker's)	1 T.	2

Food and Description	Measure or Quantity	Sodium (mgs.)
RAVIOLI:		
Canned, regular pack (Franco-American):		
Beef, *RavioliOs*	7½-oz. serving	1030
Cheese, in tomato sauce, *RavioliOs*	7½-oz. can	1160
Canned, dietetic (Featherweight) beef	8-oz. can	68
RELISH, sweet (Smucker's)	1 T.	158
RENNET MIX (Junket):		
*Powder:		
Chocolate, made with whole milk	½ cup	65
Vanilla, made with skim milk	½ cup	70
Tablet	1 tablet	165
RHINE WINE:		
(Gold Seal)	3 fl. oz.	3
(Great Western)	3 fl. oz.	25
RHUBARB, cooked, sweetened	½ cup	2
RICE:		
*Brown (Uncle Ben's) parboiled, with butter & salt	⅔ cup	458
*White:		
(Minute Rice) instant, no added butter or salt	⅔ cup	2
(Uncle Ben's) with butter & salt	⅔ cup	323
RICE, FRIED (See also RICE MIX):		
*Canned (La Choy)	⅓ of 11-oz. can	966
Frozen:		
(Birds Eye)	3.7 oz.	429
(La Choy) & pork	6-oz. serving	1716
*RICE, FRIED, SEASONING MIX (Durkee)	1 cup	1597
RICE KRINKLES, cereal (Post)	⅞ cup	179
RICE KRISPIES, cereal (Kellogg's):		
Regular	1 cup	285
Frosted	¾ cup	200
RICE MIX:		
*Beef (Minute Rice)	½ cup	720
*Chicken (Minute Rice)	½ cup	694
*Fried (Minute Rice)	½ cup	634
*Long grain & wild (Uncle Ben's) with added butter	½ cup	442
*Spanish (Minute Rice)	½ cup	839
RICE, SPANISH:		
Canned, regular pack:		
(Comstock)	½ of 7½-oz. can	850

Food and Description	Measure or Quantity	Sodium (mgs.)
(Libby's)	7½-oz. serving	1108
Canned, dietetic (Featherweight)	7½ oz.	32
Frozen (Birds Eye)	3.7 oz.	495
RICE & VEGETABLE, frozen:		
(Birds Eye):		
French style & peas with mushrooms	3.7 oz.	637
(Green Giant) *Rice Originals:*		
& broccoli in cheese sauce	½ cup	405
Country French style	½ cup	430
Festive	½ cup	315
Medley	½ cup	280
Pilaf	½ cup	520
Verdi	½ cup	500
ROE, baked or broiled, cod & shad	4 oz.	83
ROLL OR BUN:		
Commercial type, non-frozen:		
Biscuit (Wonder)	1 ¼-oz. piece	188
Brown & Serve (Wonder):		
Buttermilk	1-oz. piece	142
French	1-oz. piece	151
Gem style	1-oz. piece	156
Home bake	1-oz. piece	114
Commercial type, non-frozen:		
Club (Pepperidge Farm)	1⅓-oz. piece	267
Crescent (Pepperidge Farm) butter	1-oz. piece	165
Croissant (Pepperidge Farm):		
Butter	2-oz. piece	310
Chocolate	2.4-oz. piece	325
Walnut	2-oz. piece	275
Dinner:		
Home Pride	1-oz. piece	170
(Pepperidge Farm)	.7-oz. piece	95
(Wonder)	1¼-oz. piece	188
Finger (Pepperidge Farm):		
Sesame seed	.6-oz. piece	120
White poppy	.6-oz. piece	80
Frankfurter:		
(Arnold) Hot Dog	1.3-oz. piece	290
(Pepperidge Farm)	1¾-oz. piece	240
(Wonder)	2-oz. piece	153
French:		
(Arnold) *Francisco,* Sourdough	1.1-oz. piece	160

Food and Description	Measure or Quantity	Sodium (mgs.)
(Pepperidge Farm):		
Small	1⅓-oz. piece	245
Large	3-oz. piece	550
Golden Twist (Pepperidge Farm)	1-oz. piece	150
Hamburger:		
(Arnold)	1.4-oz. piece	285
(Pepperidge Farm)	1½-oz. piece	250
(Wonder)	2-oz. piece	153
Hoggie (Wonder)	6-oz. piece	869
Honey (Hostess) glazed	3¾-oz. piece	522
Kaiser (Wonder)	6-oz. piece	869
Old fashioned (Pepperidge Farm)	.6-oz. piece	95
Pan (Wonder)	1¼-oz. piece	188
Parkerhouse (Pepperidge Farm)	.6-oz. piece	95
Party (Pepperidge Farm)	.4-oz. piece	55
Sandwich (Arnold) soft, plain or sesame	1.3-oz. roll	260
Soft (Pepperidge Farm)	1¼-oz. piece	235
Sourdough French (Pepperidge Farm)	1⅓-oz. piece	255
Frozen:		
Apple crunch (Sara Lee)	1-oz. piece	105
Caramel pecan (Sara Lee)	1.3-oz. piece	148
Caramel sticky (Sara Lee)	1-oz. piece	110
Cinnamon (Sara Lee)	.9-oz. piece	96
Croissant (Sara Lee)	.9-oz. piece	140
Crumb (Sara Lee):		
Blueberry	1¾-oz. piece	191
French	1¾-oz. piece	170
Danish (Sara Lee):		
Apple	1.3-oz. piece	110
Cheese	1.3-oz. piece	124
Cherry	1.3-oz. piece	103
Cinnamon raisin	1.3-oz. piece	132
Pecan	1.3-oz. piece	119
Honey:		
(Morton):		
Regular	2¼-oz. piece	13
Mini	1.3-oz. piece	78
(Sara Lee)	1-oz. piece	119
ROLL OR BUN DOUGH:		
*Frozen (Rich's):		
Cinnamon	2¼-oz. piece	226
Frankfurter	1 piece	238
Hamburger, regular	1 piece	227
Onion, regular	1 piece	226

Food and Description	Measure or Quantity	Sodium (mgs.)
Parkerhouse	1 piece	133
Refrigerated (Pillsbury):		
Caramel danish, with nuts	1 piece	242
Cinnamon with icing, *Ballard*	1 piece	310
Cinnamon raisin danish	1 piece	225
Crescent	1 piece	665
Wheat, Bakery Style	1 piece	295
White, Bakery Style	1 piece	335
*ROLL MIX, HOT (Pillsbury)	1 piece	125
ROMAN MEAL cereal, plain	⅓ cup	2
ROSEMARY LEAVES (French's)	1 tsp.	<1
ROSE WINE (Great Western)	3 fl. oz.	38
RUTABAGA canned (Sunshine)		
solids & liq.	½ cup	393

S

Food and Description	Measure or Quantity	Sodium (mgs.)
SAGE (French's)	1 tsp.	<1
SALAD DRESSING:		
Regular:		
Bleu or blue cheese:		
(USDA)	1 T.	164
(Seven Seas) chunky	1 T.	195
(Wish-Bone) chunky	1 T.	149
Caesar (Seven Seas) *Viva*	1 T.	205
French:		
(Bernstein's) creamy	1 T.	224
(Seven Seas) creamy	1 T.	265
Garlic (Wish-Bone) creamy	1 T.	83
Green Goddess (Seven Seas)	1 T.	140
Herb & spice (Seven Seas)	1 T.	160
Italian:		
(Bernstein's)	1 T.	184
(Seven Seas) creamy	1 T.	255
(Wish-Bone)	1 T.	362
Onion 'N Chive (Seven Seas)		
creamy	1 T.	190
Roquefort (Bernstein's)	1 T.	142
Spin Blend (Hellmann's)	1 T.	112

Food and Description	Measure or Quantity	Sodium (mgs.)
Sweet 'N Sour (Dutch Pantry) creamy	1 T.	63
Thousand Island:		
(Bernstein's)	1 T.	127
(Seven Seas)	1 T.	350
Vinaigrette (Bernstein's) French	1 T.	180
Dietetic:		
Bleu or blue cheese (Walden Farms) chunky	1 T.	660
Caesar:		
(Estee) garlic	1 T.	15
(Featherweight) creamy	1 T.	16
Cucumber (Featherweight) creamy	1 T.	12
Cucumber & onion (Featherweight) creamy	1 T.	128
French:		
(Featherweight) low sodium	1 T.	4
(Walden Farms)	1 T.	330
Herb & Spice (Featherweight)	1 T.	5
Italian:		
(Estee) spicy	1 T.	12
(Featherweight)	1 T.	127
(Walden Farms) Classico	1 T.	300
Red wine/vinegar (Featherweight)	1 T.	63
Russian:		
(Featherweight) creamy	1 T.	134
(Wish-Bone)	1 T.	160
Thousand Island (Wish-Bone)	1 T.	173
2-Calorie Low Sodium (Featherweight)	1 T.	6
SALAD DRESSING MIX:		
*Regular (Good Seasons):		
Bleu or blue cheese	1 T.	228
Buttermilk Farm Style	1 T.	147
Farm Style	1 T.	124
French:		
Regular	1 T.	205
Old fashioned	1 T.	185
Garlic:		
Regular	1 T.	236
Cheese	1 T.	184
Italian:		
Regular	1 T.	184
Cheese	1 T.	188
Zesty	1 T.	131
Onion	1 T.	138

Food and Description	Measure or Quantity	Sodium (mgs.)
Dietetic:		
*Blue cheese (Weight Watchers)	1 T.	108
*French (Weight Watchers)	1 T.	164
Italian:		
*(Good Seasons)	1 T.	161
*(Weight Watchers):		
Regular	1 T.	175
Creamy	1 T.	224
*Russian (Weight Watchers)	1 T.	128
*Thousand Island (Weight Watchers)	1 T.	265
SALAMI:		
(Best's Kosher):		
Club	1-oz. serving	443
Sliced	1-oz. serving	445
(Hormel):		
Genoa, *Dilusso*	1-oz. slice	543
Hard	1-oz. slice	460
(Oscar Mayer):		
For beer	.8-oz. slice	282
For beer, beef	.8-oz. slice	234
Cotto	.8-oz. slice	245
Hard	.3-oz. slice	167
(Oscherwitz):		
Chub	1-oz. serving	443
Sliced	1-oz. serving	445
(Swift) Genoa	1-oz. serving	642
SALISBURY STEAK:		
Canned (Morton House)	6¼-oz. serving	512
Frozen:		
(Banquet):		
Buffet Supper	2-lb. pkg.	5518
Dinner	11-oz. dinner	2059
Man Pleaser	19-oz. dinner	3741
(Green Giant):		
With gravy, baked	7 oz.	1177
With creole sauce, *Boil 'N Bag*	9 oz.	910
(Stouffer's) with onion gravy	6 oz.	1150
(Swanson):		
Regular, with gravy	10-oz. entree	1435
Hungry Man	17-oz. dinner	1800
3-course	16-oz. dinner	1835
TV Brand	11½-oz. dinner	1345
SALMON:		
Canned, regular pack:		
Keta (Bumble Bee) solids & liq.	½ cup	536

Food and Description	Measure or Quantity	Sodium (mgs.)
Pink or Humpback:		
(Bumble Bee) solids & liq.	½ cup	542
(Del Monte)	7¾-oz. can	1220
Sockeye or Red or Blueback:		
(Bumble Bee) solids & liq.	½ cup	455
(Del Monte)	7¾-oz. can	1169
Canned, dietetic (S&W) *Nutradiet*, low sodium	½ cup	45
SALT:		
Regular:		
Regular (USDA)	1 tsp.	2132
Lite (Morton)	1 tsp.	1188
Butter flavor (French's)	1 tsp.	1090
Hickory smoke (French's)	1 tsp.	1170
Substitute:		
(Adolph's) regular or seasoned	1 tsp.	<1
(Morton) regular or seasoned	1 tsp.	<1
SANDWICH SPREAD:		
(Hellmann's)	1 T.	191
(Oscar Mayer)	1-oz. serving	279
SARDINE, canned:		
Atlantic (Del Monte) with tomato sauce	7½-oz. can	827
Imported (Underwood) in mustard or tomato sauce	3¾-oz. can	850
Norwegian (Underwood) in oil	3¾-oz. can	850
SAUCE:		
Regular pack:		
A-1	1 T.	275
Barbecue:		
Chris & Pitt's	1 T.	141
(French's) regular	1 T.	255
Open Pit (General Foods):		
Original	1 T.	236
Smoke flavor	1 T.	232
Chili (See CHILI SAUCE)		
Escoffier Sauce Diable	1 T.	160
Escoffier Sauce Robert	1 T.	70
Famous Sauce	1 T.	67
Hot, *Frank's*	1 tsp.	131
Italian (Contadina)	4 fl. oz.	601
Salsa Mexicana (Contadina)	4 fl. oz.	570
Salsa Picante (Del Monte)	¼ cup	405
Salsa Roja (Del Monte)	¼ cup	509
Seafood cocktail (Del Monte)	1 T.	228
Soy:		
(Kikkoman)	1 T.	932

Food and Description	Measure or Quantity	Sodium (mgs.)
(La Choy)	1 T.	974
Steak (Dawn Fresh) with mushrooms	1-oz. serving	300
Steak Supreme	1 T.	125
Sweet & sour:		
(Contadina)	1 oz.	96
(La Choy)	1-oz. serving	222
Taco:		
(Del Monte):		
Hot	¼ cup	439
Mild	¼ cup	481
(Ortega)	1 T.	80
Tartar (Hellmann's)	1 T.	182
Teriyaki (Kikkoman)	1 T.	622
V-8	1-oz. serving	270
White, medium	¼ cup	242
Worcestershire (French's) regular or smoky	1 T.	165
SAUCE MIX:		
Regular:		
A la King (Durkee)	1-oz. pkg.	1384
*Cheese:		
(Durkee)	½ cup	446
(French's)	½ cup	850
Hollandaise:		
(Durkee)	1-oz. pkg.	548
*(French's)	1 T.	97
Sour cream:		
*(Durkee)	⅔ cup	727
*(French's)	2½ T.	130
*Stroganoff (French's)	⅓ cup	490
*Sweet & sour (Durkee)	1 cup	1053
*Teriyaki (French's)	1 T.	593
*White (Durkee)	1 cup	696
Dietetic (Weight Watchers) lemon butter	1 pkg.	1895
SAUERKRAUT:		
(Claussen) drained	½ cup	506
(Del Monte) solids & liq.	1 cup	1468
(Silver Floss) any type	½ cup	750
SAUSAGE:		
Brown 'n Serve (Swift) original	.8-oz. link	169
Italian-Style (Best's Kosher; Oscherwitz)	3-oz. piece	1107
Polish-style (Frito-Lay) beef, smoked	1 oz.	525

Food and Description	Measure or Quantity	Sodium (mgs.)
(Best's Kosher; Oscherwitz)	3-oz. piece	1193
Pork:		
(Jimmy Dean)	2-oz. serving	338
*(Oscar Mayer) *Little Friers*	.6-oz. link	223
Smoked:		
(Best's Kosher; Oscherwitz)	3-oz. piece	1193
(Hormel) pork	3-oz. serving	1059
(Oscar Mayer) beef	1½-oz. link	455
SAUSAGE SANDWICH, frozen (Stouffer's)	8¼ oz.	1838
SAUTERNE, (Great Western)	3 fl. oz.	34
SCALLOP:		
Steamed	4-oz. serving	301
Frozen (Mrs. Paul's) with butter & cheese	7-oz.pkg.	1330
SEAFOOD PLATTER, frozen (Mrs. Paul's) breaded, fried	4½-oz. serving	1080
SEAFOOD SEASONING (French's)	1 tsp.	1410
SEAWEED:		
Raw, Irishmars	1 oz.	822
Dried, Agar	1 oz.	33
SELTZER (Canada Dry)	6 fl. oz.	<10
SESAME SEEDS (French's)	1 tsp.	<1
SHAD, CREOLE	4-oz. serving	83
SHAKE 'N BAKE:		
Chicken, original	1 pkg.	2363
Crispy country mild	1 pkg.	2041
Fish	2-oz. pkg.	1049
Italian	1 pkg.	2098
Pork:		
Original	1 pkg.	2541
Barbecue	1 pkg.	2644
SHERRY:		
Cocktail (Gold Seal)	3 fl. oz.	3
Cream (Great Western) Solera	3 fl. oz.	32
Dry (Great Western) Solera	3 fl. oz.	34
SHREDDED WHEAT (Quaker)	1 piece	<1
SHRIMP:		
Raw, meat only	4 oz.	159
Frozen (Mrs. Paul's) fried	3-oz. serving	480
SHRIMP DINNER, frozen (Van de Kamp's)	10 oz.	880
SLENDER (Carnation):		
Bar:		
Chocolate or chocolate peanut butter	1 bar	142

Food and Description	Measure or Quantity	Sodium (mgs.)
Chocolate chip	1 bar	157
Lemon raspberry or strawberry yogurt	1 bar	137
Vanilla	1 bar	160
Dry:		
Chocolate	1 packet	200
Dutch chocolate or French vanilla	1 packet	110
Lemon yogurt	1 packet	75
Liquid:		
Banana, peach or strawberry	10-fl.-oz. can	430
Chocolate	10-fl.-oz. can	515
Chocolate fudge or vanilla	10-fl.-oz. can	550
SLOPPY HOT DOG SEASONING MIX (French's)	1½-oz. pkg.	220
SLOPPY JOE:		
Canned (Morton House) beef	5 oz.	2758
Frozen (Banquet) *Cookin' Bag*	5-oz. bag	903
SLOPPY JOE SEASONING MIX:		
*(Durkee):		
Regular flavor	1¼ cups	1788
Pizza flavor	1¼ cups	1515
(French's)	1½-oz. pkg.	3120
SNACK BAR (Pepperidge Farm):		
Apple nut, apricot-raspberry, blueberry or date nut	1 piece	90
Brownie nut	1 piece	100
Chocolate chip & coconut macaroons or raisin spice	1 piece	80
SNO BALL (Hostess)	1 cake	170
SOFT DRINK:		
Sweetened:		
Birch beer (Canada Dry)	6 fl. oz.	14
Bitter lemon:		
(Canada Dry)	6 fl. oz.	13
(Schweppes)	6 fl. oz.	2
Bubble Up	6 fl. oz.	16
Cactus Cooler (Canada Dry)	6 fl. oz.	16
Cherry:		
(Canada Dry) wild	6 fl. oz.	16
(Shasta) black	6 fl. oz.	18
Club:		
(Canada Dry)	6 fl. oz.	39
(Shasta)	6 fl. oz.	11
Cola:		
Coca-Cola:		
Regular	6 fl. oz.	7

Food and Description	Measure or Quantity	Sodium (mgs.)
Caffeine-free	6 fl. oz.	3
Pepsi-Cola, regular or *Pepsi Free*	6 fl. oz.	5
(Royal Crown)	6 fl. oz.	Tr.
(Shasta)	6 fl. oz.	22
Collins mix (Canada Dry)	6 fl. oz.	13
Cream:		
(Canada Dry) vanilla	6 fl. oz.	14
(Schweppes) red	6 fl. oz.	15
(Shasta)	6 fl. oz.	12
Dr. Pepper	6 fl. oz.	9
Fruit Punch:		
(Nehi)	6 fl. oz.	8
(Shasta)	6 fl. oz.	15
Ginger ale:		
(Canada Dry) regular	6 fl. oz.	5
(Fanta)	6 fl. oz.	14
(Nehi)	6 fl. oz.	Tr.
(Schweppes)	6 fl. oz.	11
(Shasta)	6 fl. oz.	11
Ginger beer (Schweppes)	6 fl. oz.	14
Grape:		
(Canada Dry) concord	6 fl. oz.	16
(Fanta)	6 fl. oz.	7
(Hi-C)	6 fl. oz.	6
(Nehi)	6 fl. oz.	8
(Patio)	6 fl. oz.	21
(Schweppes)	6 fl. oz.	15
Half & half (Canada Dry)	6 fl. oz.	13
Hi-Spot (Canada Dry)	6 fl. oz.	19
Island Lime (Canada Dry)	6 fl. oz.	14
Lemon-line (Shasta)	6 fl. oz.	28
Mello Yello	6 fl. oz.	14
Mountain Dew	6 fl. oz.	16
Mr. PiBB	6 fl. oz.	10
Orange:		
(Canada Dry) *Sunripe*	6 fl. oz.	16
(Fanta)	6 fl. oz.	7
(Hi-C)	6 fl. oz.	7
(Nehi)	6 fl. oz.	11
(Patio)	6 fl. oz.	21
(Shasta)	6 fl. oz.	15
Peach (Nehi)	6 fl. oz.	16
Pineapple (Canada Dry)	6 fl. oz.	16
Punch (Hi-C)	6 fl. oz.	6
Quinine or Tonic Water:		
(Canada Dry)	6 fl. oz.	5

Food and Description	Measure or Quantity	Sodium (mgs.)
(Schweppes)	6 fl. oz.	4
Rondo (Schweppes)	6 fl. oz.	13
Root Beer:		
Barrelhead (Canada Dry)	6 fl. oz.	13
(Dad's)	6 fl. oz.	14
(Fanta)	6 fl. oz.	10
(Nehi)	6 fl. oz.	9
On Tap	6 fl. oz.	9
(Patio)	6 fl. oz.	2
Rooti (Canada Dry)	6 fl. oz.	13
(Shasta) draft	6 fl. oz.	13
Seven-Up	6 fl. oz.	16
Sprite	6 fl. oz.	23
Strawberry:		
(Canada Dry) California	6 fl. oz.	16
(Nehi)	6 fl. oz. (from can)	7
(Shasta)	6 fl. oz.	23
Tahitian Treat (Canada Dry)	6 fl. oz.	16
Teem	6 fl. oz.	16
Upper 10 (Royal Crown)	6 fl. oz.	20
Whiskey sour (Canada Dry)	6 fl. oz.	13
Wink (Canada Dry)	6 fl. oz.	14
Dietetic or low calorie:		
Bubble Up	6 fl. oz.	48
Cherry:		
(No-Cal)	6 fl. oz.	44
(Shasta) black	6 fl. oz.	24
Chocolate (No-Cal)	6 fl. oz.	33
Coffee (Canada Dry)	6 fl. oz.	45
Cola:		
(Canada Dry)	6 fl. oz.	20
Coca-Cola, regular or caffeine free	6 fl. oz.	16
Diet-Rite	6 fl. oz.	19
(No-Cal)	6 fl. oz.	18
Pepsi:		
Diet	6 fl. oz.	31
Free	6 fl. oz.	35
Light	6 fl. oz.	21
(Shasta) regular or cherry	6 fl. oz.	22
Cream:		
(No-Cal)	6 fl. oz.	33
(Shasta)	6 fl. oz.	25
Dr. Pepper	6 fl. oz.	Tr.
Fresca	6 fl. oz.	18

Food and Description	Measure or Quantity	Sodium (mgs.)
Ginger Ale:		
(Canada Dry)	6 fl. oz.	22
(No-Cal)	6 fl. oz.	30
(Shasta)	6 fl. oz.	18
Grape (Shasta)	6 fl. oz.	30
Grapefruit (Shasta)	6 fl. oz.	25
Lemon-lime (No-Cal)	6 fl. oz.	29
Mr. PiBB	6 fl. oz.	19
Orange:		
(Canada Dry)	6 fl. oz.	19
(No-Cal)	6 fl. oz.	19
(Shasta)	6 fl. oz.	26
Quinine or Tonic (No-Cal)	6 fl. oz.	15
RC 100 (Royal Crown)	6 fl. oz.	19
Root Beer:		
Barrelhead (Canada Dry)	6 fl. oz.	19
(Dad's)	6 fl. oz.	41
(No-Cal)	6 fl. oz.	30
(Ramblin')	6 fl. oz.	29
(Shasta) draft	6 fl. oz.	27
Seven-Up	6 fl. oz.	24
Sprite	6 fl. oz.	22
Strawberry (Shasta)	6 fl. oz.	25
Tab	6 fl. oz.	15
SOLE, frozen:		
(Mrs. Paul's) fillets, with lemon butter	4½-oz. serving	808
(Van de Kamp's) batter dipped, french fried	1 piece	289
(Weight Watchers) in lemon sauce	9¼-oz. meal	1180
SOUFFLE (Stouffer's) cheese	6-oz. serving	1360
SOUP:		
Canned, regular pack:		
*Asparagus (Campbell) condensed, cream of	8 oz.	980
Bean (Campbell):		
Chunky, with ham, old fashioned	11-oz. can	1400
*Condensed, with bacon	8 oz.	990
*Semi-condensed, *Soup For One,* with ham	11 oz.	1480
Bean, black:		
*(Campbell) condensed	8 oz.	1125
(Crosse & Blackwell)	6½ oz.	757

Food and Description	Measure or Quantity	Sodium (mgs.)
Beef:		
(Campbell):		
Chunky:		
Regular	10¾-oz. can	1280
With noodles	10¾-oz. can	1500
*Condensed:		
Regular	8 oz.	950
Broth:		
Plain	8 oz.	940
& barley	8 oz.	980
& noodles	8 oz.	900
Consomme	8 oz.	900
Mushroom	8 oz.	1110
Noodle	8 oz.	990
Teriyaki	8 oz.	960
(Swanson)	7½-oz. can	840
Celery:		
*(Campbell) condensed, cream of	8 oz.	940
*(Rokeach) condensed:		
Prepared with milk	10 oz.	1020
Prepared with water	10 oz.	950
*Cheddar cheese (Campbell)	8 oz.	930
Chicken:		
(Campbell):		
Chunky:		
Regular	10¾-oz. can	1290
Old fashioned	10¾-oz. can	1410
& rice	19-oz. can	2400
Vegetable	19-oz. can	2520
*Condensed:		
Alphabet	8 oz.	950
Broth:		
Plain	8 oz.	860
& rice	8 oz.	960
Cream of	8 oz.	950
Gumbo	8 oz.	930
Mushroom, creamy	8 oz.	980
NoodleOs	8 oz.	890
Oriental	8 oz.	970
& rice	8 oz.	890
Vegetable	8 oz.	930
*Semi-condensed, *Soup For One:*		
& noodles, golden	11 oz.	1510
Vegetable, full flavored	11 oz.	1550

Food and Description	Measure or Quantity	Sodium (mgs.)
(Swanson) broth	7¼-oz. can	960
Chili beef (Campbell):		
Chunky	11-oz. can	1370
*Condensed	8 oz.	980
Chowder:		
Clam:		
Manhattan style:		
(Campbell):		
Chunky	18-oz. can	2520
*Condensed	8 oz.	940
(Crosse & Blackwell)	6½ oz.	803
New England style:		
*(Campbell):		
Condensed:		
Made with milk	8 oz.	1020
Made with water	8 oz.	965
Semi-condensed, *Soup For One:*		
Made with milk	11 oz.	1480
Made with water	11 oz.	1420
(Crosse & Blackwell)	6½-oz.	637
Consomme madrilene (Crosse & Blackwell)	6½ oz.	609
Crab (Crosse & Blackwell)	6½ oz.	933
Gazpacho:		
*(Campbell's) condensed	8 oz.	630
(Crosse & Blackwell)	6½ oz.	1653
Ham'n butter bean (Campbell)		
Chunky	10¾-oz. can	1430
Lentil (Crosse & Blackwell) with ham	6½ oz.	979
*Meatball alphabet (Campbell) condensed	8 oz.	1025
Mexicali bean (Campbell)		
Chunky	19½-oz. can	2160
Minestrone:		
(Campbell):		
Chunky	18-oz. can	2660
*Condensed	8 oz.	960
(Crosse & Blackwell)	6½ oz.	720
Mushroom:		
*(Campbell):		
Condensed:		
Cream of	8 oz.	870
Golden	8 oz.	960

Food and Description	Measure or Quantity	Sodium (mgs.)
Semi-condensed, *Soup For One*, cream of, savory	11 oz.	1560
(Crosse & Blackwell) cream of, bisque	6½ oz.	923
*(Rokeach) cream of:		
Prepared with milk	10 oz.	1170
Prepared with water	10 oz.	1050
*Mushroom barley (Campbell's)	8 oz.	970
*Noodle (Campbell):		
Curly noodle with chicken	8 oz.	1025
& ground beef	8 oz.	850
*Onion (Campbell):		
Regular	8 oz.	990
Cream of:		
Made with water	8 oz.	910
Made with water & milk	8 oz.	940
*Oyster stew (Campbell):		
Made with milk	8 oz.	1040
Made with water	8 oz.	985
*Pea, green (Campbell)	8 oz.	900
Pea, split (Campbell):		
Chunky, with ham	18-oz. can	2420
*Condensed, with ham & bacon	8 oz.	850
*Pepper pot (Campbell)	8 oz.	1065
*Potato (Campbell) cream of:		
Made with water	8 oz.	960
Made with water & milk	8 oz.	990
*Scotch broth (Campbell)	8 oz.	950
Shrimp:		
*(Campbell) condensed, cream of:		
Made with milk	8 oz.	1020
Made with water	8 oz.	970
(Crosse & Blackwell) cream of	6½ oz.	1459
Sirloin burger (Campbell) *Chunky*	19-oz. can	2500
Steak & potato (Campbell) *Chunky*	19-oz. can	2740
Tomato:		
*(Campbell):		
Condensed:		
Regular:		
Made with milk	8 oz.	810
Made with water	8 oz.	760
Bisque	8 oz.	980
& rice, old fashioned	8 oz.	810

Food and Description	Measure or Quantity	Sodium (mgs.)
Semi-condensed, *Soup For One*, Royale	11 oz.	1320
*(Rokeach):		
Made with milk	10 oz.	1059
Made with water	10 oz.	980
Turkey (Campbell):		
Chunky	18¾-oz. can	2580
*Condensed:		
Noodle	8 oz.	970
Vegetable	8 oz.	910
Vegetable:		
(Campbell):		
Chunky:		
Regular	19-oz. can	2600
Beef, old fashioned	19-oz. can	2360
Mediterranean	19-oz. can	2420
*Condensed:		
Regular	8 oz.	770
Beef	8 oz.	880
Vegetarian	8 oz.	790
*Semi-condensed, *Soup For One:*		
Barley, with beef	11 oz.	1600
Old world	11 oz.	1530
*(Rokeach) vegetarian	10 oz.	1055
Vichyssoise (Crosse & Blackwell) cream of	6½ oz.	702
*Won ton (Campbell)	8 oz.	890
Canned, dietetic pack:		
Beef (Campbell) & mushroom, low sodium	10¾-oz. can	75
Chicken:		
(Campbell) low sodium:		
Chunky	7½-oz. can	70
With noodles	10¾-oz. can	100
Vegetable	10¾-oz. can	100
*(Dia-Mel) broth	8 oz.	10
Corn (Campbell) low sodium	10¾-oz. can	55
Mushroom (Campbell) cream of low sodium	7¼-oz. can	35
Pea, green (Campbell) low sodium	7½-oz. can	30
Pea, split (Campbell) low sodium	10¾-oz. can	25
Tomato (Campbell) low sodium:		
Regular	7¼-oz. can	40
With tomato pieces	10½-oz. can	90

Food and Description	Measure or Quantity	Sodium (mgs.)
Turkey (Campbell) & noodle, low sodium	7¼-oz. can	50
Vegetable (Campbell) low sodium:		
Regular	7¼-oz. can	50
Chunky	10¾-oz. can	75
Frozen:		
*Barley & mushroom (Mother's Own)	8 oz.	490
Chowder, Clam, New England style (Stouffer's)	8 oz.	508
Pea, split:		
*(Mother's Own)	8 oz.	575
(Stouffer's)	8¼ oz.	694
Spinach (Stouffer's) cream of	8 oz.	883
*Vegetable (Mother's Own)	8 oz.	560
*Won ton (La Choy)	1 cup	2027
Mix:		
*Beef (Weight Watchers) broth	6 fl. oz.	1042
SOUP GREENS (Durkee)	2½-oz. jar	408
SOYBEAN CURD or TOFU	2¾″ × 1½″ × 1″ cake	8
SPAGHETTI:		
Cooked:		
8-10 minutes, "Al Dente"	1 cup	1
14-20 minutes, tender	1 cup	1
Canned:		
(Franco-American):		
With little meatballs in tomato sauce	7⅜-oz. can	1040
With meatballs in tomato sauce, *SpaghettiOs*	7⅜-oz. can	1060
In meat sauce	7½-oz. can	1130
With sliced franks in tomato sauce, *SpaghettiOs*	7⅜-oz. can	1070
In tomato sauce with cheese	7⅜-oz. can	940
(Libby's) & meatballs in tomato sauce	7½-oz. serving	1359
Dietetic (Featherweight) & meatballs	7½-oz. serving	95
Frozen:		
(Banquet):		
Buffet Supper, & meatballs	2-lb. pkg.	5336
Dinner, & meatballs	11½-oz. dinner	1851
Entree, with meat sauce	8-oz. entree	1426
(Green Giant) & meatballs in tomato sauce	9-oz. entree	989
(Morton) & meatballs	11-oz. dinner	911

Food and Description	Measure or Quantity	Sodium (mgs.)
(Stouffer's) & meat sauce	14-oz. pkg.	1970
(Swanson) *TV Brand*	12½-oz. dinner	1065
SPAGHETTI SAUCE:		
Canned, regular pack:		
Marinara (Prince)	4-oz. serving	590
Meat or meat flavored:		
(Prego)	4-oz. serving	810
(Prince)	½ cup	626
Meatless or plain:		
(Prego)	4-oz. serving	790
(Prince)	½ cup	732
Mushroom:		
(Prego)	4-oz. serving	670
(Prince)	4-oz. serving	580
Canned, dietetic pack		
(Featherweight)	⅔ cup	<10
*SPAGHETTI SAUCE MIX:		
(Durkee) plain	½ cup	747
(French's):		
Italian style	⅝ cup	900
Thick, homemade style	⅞ cup	1455
***SPAM,* luncheon meat (Hormel):**		
Regular	1-oz. serving	341
With cheese chunks	1-oz. serving	341
Deviled	1-oz. serving	361
***SPECIAL K,* cereal (Kellogg's)**	1 cup	225
SPINACH:		
Fresh, whole leaves	½ cup	16
Boiled	½ cup	39
Canned, regular pack, solids & liq.:		
(Del Monte)	½ cup	372
(Sunshine)	½ cup	300
Frozen:		
(Birds Eye):		
Chopped	⅓ of pkg.	69
Creamed	⅓ of pkg.	277
Leaf	⅓ of pkg.	77
(Green Giant):		
Creamed	⅓ of pkg.	332
Cut, in butter sauce	⅓ of pkg.	309
Harvest Fresh	4 oz.	318
(McKenzie):		
Chopped	3⅓ oz.	70
Cut leaf	3⅓ oz.	77
(Stouffer's) souffle	4 oz.	600

111

Food and Description	Measure or Quantity	Sodium (mgs.)
SQUASH, SUMMER:		
Yellow, boiled slices	½ cup	<1
Zucchini, boiled slices	½ cup	<1
Canned (Del Monte) zucchini in tomato sauce	½ cup	424
Frozen:		
(Birds Eye) zucchini	3⅓ oz.	2
(McKenzie) Crookneck	⅓ of pkg.	1
(Mrs. Paul's) sticks, batter fried	⅓ of pkg.	630
SQUASH, WINTER:		
Acorn, baked	½ cup	1
Hubbard, baked, mashed	½ cup	1
Frozen:		
(Birds Eye)	⅓ of pkg.	2
(Southland) butternut	4 oz.	2
STEAK & GREEN PEPPERS, frozen:		
(Green Giant):	9-oz. entree	1222
(Swanson)	8½-oz. entree	1105
STOCK BASE (French's) beef or chicken	1 tsp.	480
STRAWBERRY:		
Fresh, capped	½ cup	<1
Frozen (Birds Eye):		
Halves	⅓ of pkg.	1
Whole	¼ of pkg.	<1
Whole, quick thaw	½ of pkg.	6
STRAWBERRY DRINK (Hi-C):		
Canned	6 fl. oz.	<1
*Mix	6 fl. oz.	43
STRAWBERRY NECTAR (Libby's)	6 fl. oz.	5
STRAWBERRY PRESERVE OR JAM:		
Sweetened (Smucker's)	1 T.	2
Dietetic or low calorie (See Strawberry Spread)		
STRAWBERRY SHORTCAKE, cereal (General Mills)	1 cup	190
STRAWBERRY SPREAD, dietetic:		
(Diet Delight)	1 T.	30
(Estee)	1 T.	Tr.
(Featherweight) artificially sweetened	1 T.	45
STUFFING MIX:		
*Beef, *Stove Top*	½ cup	528
*Chicken, *Stove Top*	½ cup	638
*Cornbread, *Stove Top*	½ cup	552

Food and Description	Measure or Quantity	Sodium (mgs.)
Cube (Pepperidge Farm)	1 oz.	510
Herb seasoned (Pepperidge Farm)	1 oz.	520
*Pork, Stove Top	½ cup	616
*San Francisco Style Stove Top	½ cup	637
Seasoned (Pepperidge Farm)	1 oz.	510
White bread, Mrs. Cubbison's	1 oz.	480
SUCCOTASH:		
Canned:		
(Libby's) cream style	½ cup	317
(Stokely-Van Camp)	½ cup	275
Frozen (Birds Eye)	⅓ of pkg.	35
SUGAR:		
Brown	1 T.	4
Confectioners'	1 T.	<1
Granulated	1 T.	<1
Maple	1¾" × 1¼" × ½" piece	4
***SUGAR CORN POPS,** cereal (Kellogg's)	1 cup	95
***SUGAR CRISP,** cereal	⅞ cup	25
***SUGAR PUFFS,** cereal (Malt-O-Meal)	⅞ cup	26
***SUGAR SMACKS,** cereal (Kellogg's)	¾ cup	70
SUGAR SUBSTITUTE:		
(Featherweight)	3 drops	5
Sprinkle Sweet (Pillsbury)	1 tsp.	1
SWEET *10 (Pillsbury)	⅛ tsp.	2
***SUNFLOWER SEED** (Fisher):		
In hull, roasted, salted	1 oz.	58
Hulled, dry roasted, salted	1 oz.	108
Hulled, oil roasted, salted	1 oz.	108
***SUZY Q** (Hostess):		
Banana	1 cake	195
Chocolate	1 cake	313
SWEET POTATO:		
Baked, peeled	5" × 1" potato	13
Canned, heavy syrup	4-oz. serving	54
Frozen (Mrs. Paul's) candied, with apple	4-oz. serving	320
***SWEET & SOUR ORIENTAL,** canned (La Choy):		
Chicken	7½-oz. serving	1335
Pork	7½-oz. serving	1455
SWISS STEAK, frozen (Swanson) TV Brand	10-oz. dinner	775

Food and Description	Measure or Quantity	Sodium (mgs.)
SYRUP (See also TOPPING):		
Regular:		
Apricot (Smucker's)	1 T.	5
Blackberry (Smucker's)	1 T.	2
Chocolate or chocolate-flavored		
Bosco	1 T.	25
(Hershey's)	1 T.	14
Corn, Karo, dark or light	1 T.	37
Maple, Karo, imitation	1 T.	32
Pancake or waffle:		
(Aunt Jemima)	1 T.	15
Golden Griddle	1 T.	20
Karo	1 T.	32
Log Cabin, regular	1 T.	6
Mrs. Butterworth's	1 T.	24
Strawberry (Smucker's)	1 T.	2
Dietetic or low calorie:		
Blueberry (Featherweight)	1 T.	<25
Chocolate-flavored (Diet Delight)	1 T.	10
Pancake or waffle:		
(Aunt Jemima)	1 T.	29
(Diet Delight)	1 T.	30
(Featherweight)	1 T.	<25

T

TACO:		
*(Ortega)	1 taco	420
*Mix (Durkee)	½ cup	558
Shell (Ortega)	1 shell	55
TAMALE:		
Canned (Hormel) beef	3¾ oz.	627
Frozen (Hormel) beef	1 tamale	618
*TANG:		
Grape	6 fl. oz.	5
Grapefruit or orange	6 fl. oz.	1
TANGERINE or MANDARIN ORANGE:		
Fresh (Sunkist)	1 large tangerine	2
Canned, regular pack (Del Monte) solids & liq.	5½-oz. serving	9

114

Food and Description	Measure or Quantity	Sodium (mgs.)
Canned, dietetic:		
(Diet Delight) juice pack	½ cup	5
(Featherweight) water pack	½ cup	<10
TANGERINE DRINK, canned (Hi-C)	6 fl. oz.	<1
*TANGERINE JUICE, frozen (Minute Maid)	6 fl. oz.	2
TAPIOCA, dry, *Minute*, quick cookies	1 T.	<1
TAQUITO, frozen (Van de Kamp's) beef	8 oz.	771
TARRAGON (French's)	1 tsp.	1
TASTEEOS, cereal (Ralston Purina)	1¼ cups	210
*TEA MIX, iced **Nestea*, lemon-flavored	8 fl. oz.	10
TERIYAKI, frozen (Stouffer's)	10 oz.	1450
*TEXTURED VEGETABLE PROTEIN, *Morningstar Farms*:		
Breakfast link	1 link	199
Breakfast patties	1 patty	409
Breakfast strips	1 strip	99
Grillers	1 patty	284
THURINGER:		
(Best's Kosher; Oscherwitz)	1-oz. serving	227
(Hormel) *Old Smokehouse*	1-oz. serving	372
(Oscar Mayer) beef	.8-oz. slice	317
TIGER TAILS (Hostess)	1 piece	249
TOASTER CAKE OR PASTRY:		
Pop-Tarts (Kellogg's):		
Regular:		
Blueberry	1 pastry	220
Brown sugar cinnamon	1 pastry	215
Chocolate chip	1 pastry	255
Frosted:		
Blueberry	1 pastry	220
Brown sugar cinnamon	1 pastry	205
Cherry	1 pastry	230
Chocolate fudge	1 pastry	255
Chocolate vanilla creme	1 pastry	285
Concord grape, dutch apple, raspberry or strawberry	1 pastry	215
Toast-R-Cake (Thomas'):		
Blueberry	1 piece	283
Bran	1 piece	316
Corn	1 piece	332
TOASTIES, cereal (Post)	1¼ cup	223

Food and Description	Measure or Quantity	Sodium (mgs.)
TOASTY O's, cereal (Malt-O-Meal)	1¼ cups	281
TOMATO:		
Regular, whole	1 med. tomato	4
Canned, regular pack:		
(Contadina):		
Sliced	½ cup	330
Whole, pear shape	½ cup	220
(Del Monte) stewed	4 oz.	381
Canned, dietetic pack:		
(Diet Delight)	½ cup	15
(Featherweight)	½ cup	<10
(S&W) *Nutradiet,* whole	½ cup	15
TOMATO JUICE:		
Canned, regular pack:		
(Campbell)	6-fl.-oz. can	660
(Del Monte)	6-fl.-oz. can	478
(Libby's)	6 fl. oz.	455
Canned, dietetic pack:		
(Diet Delight)	6 fl. oz.	20
(Featherweight)	6 fl. oz.	<20
TOMATO JUICE COCKTAIL:		
(Ocean Spray) *Firehouse Jubilee*	6 fl. oz.	599
Snap-E-Tom	6 fl. oz.	745
Regular pack:		
(Contadina) Italian	6 oz.	1800
(Del Monte)	6-oz. can	24
(Hunt's)	6-oz. can	648
Dietetic (Featherweight) low sodium	6-oz. can	70
TOMATO & PEPPER, HOT CHILI		
(Ortega) Jalapeno	1-oz. serving	119
TOMATO, PICKLED (Claussen)		
green	1 piece	336
TOMATO PUREE, canned:		
Regular (Contadina) heavy	1 cup	80
Dietetic (Featherweight)	1 cup	<20
TOMATO SAUCE, canned:		
(Contadina) regular	1 cup	1360
(Del Monte):		
Regular	1 cup	1192
Hot	1 cup	1358
With tomato tidbits	1 cup	994
TONGUE, beef, braised	4-oz. serving	69
TOPPING:		
Regular:		
Butterscotch (Smucker's)	1 T.	46
Caramel (Smucker's)	1 T.	55

Food and Description	Measure or Quantity	Sodium (mgs.)
Chocolate fudge (Hershey's)	1 T.	16
Pecans in syrup (Smucker's)	1 T.	Tr.
Pineapple (Smucker's)	1 T.	6
TOPPING, WHIPPED:		
Regular:		
Cool Whip (Birds Eye)	1 T.	2
Lucky Whip, aerosol	1 T.	4
Whip Topping (Rich's)	¼ oz.	5
Dietetic (Featherweight)	1 T.	<1
*Mix:		
Regular (Dream Whip)	1 T.	4
Dietetic (D-Zerta)	1 T.	6
TOSTADA, frozen (Van de Kamp's)	8½ oz.	1150
TOTAL, cereal:		
Regular	1 cup	375
Corn	1 cup	310
TRIPE, canned (Libby's)	6-oz. serving	147
TRIX, cereal (General Mills)	1 cup	170
TUNA:		
Canned in oil:		
(Bumble Bee):		
Chunk, light undrained	6½-oz. can	327
Solids, white undrained	7-oz. can	414
(Chicken of the Sea) chunk, light, solids & liq.	6½-oz. can	1196
Canned in water:		
(Bumble Bee):		
Chunk, light, solids & liq.	6½-oz. can	622
Solid, white, solids & liq.	7-oz. can	666
(Featherweight) light, chunk	6½ oz.	93
***TUNA HELPER** (General Mills):		
Country dumplings	⅕ of pkg.	1020
Creamy noodle	⅕ of pkg.	880
Noodles & cheese sauce	⅕ of pkg.	745
TUNA NOODLE CASSEROLE, frozen (Stouffer's)	5¾-oz. serving	670
TUNA PIE, frozen:		
(Banquet)	8-oz. pie	958
(Morton)	8-oz. pie	1120
TUNA SALAD, canned (Carnation)	1½-oz. serving	268
TURKEY:		
Canned:		
(Hormel) chunk	6 ¾-oz. serving	1128
Packaged (Oscar Mayer) breast	¾-oz. slice	295

Food and Description	Measure or Quantity	Sodium (mgs.)
Roasted:		
Dark meat	2½″ × 1⅝″ × ¼″ slice	21
Light meat	4″ × 2″ ¼″ slice	35
TURKEY DINNER OR ENTREE,		
frozen:		
(Banquet):		
Regular	11-oz. dinner	1797
Man Pleaser	19-oz. dinner	3649
(Green Giant)	9-oz. entree	366
(Swanson):		
Regular, with gravy & dressing	9¼-oz. entree	1285
Hungry Man	18-oz. dinner	2045
TV Brand	11½-oz. dinner	1200
(Weight Watchers) sliced,		
3-compartment	15¼-oz. meal	1968
TURKEY PIE, frozen:		
(Banquet):		
Regular	8-oz. pie	1017
Supreme	8-oz. pie	1370
(Morton)	8-oz. pie	1114
(Stouffer's)	10-oz. pie	1735
(Swanson):		
Regular	8-oz. pie	830
Hungry Man	1-lb. pie	1730
TURKEY TETRAZINI, frozen		
(Weight Watchers)	13-oz. bag	1441
TUMERIC (French's)	1 tsp.	<1
TURNIP GREENS:		
Canned (Sunshine) & diced turnips	½ cup	391
Frozen:		
(Birds Eye) chopped	3⅓ oz.	11
(Southland) chopped	3.2-oz.	11
TURNOVER:		
Frozen (Pepperidge Farm):		
Apple	1 turnover	215
Blueberry	1 turnover	235
Cherry	1 turnover	310
Peach	1 turnover	260
Raspberry	1 turnover	265
Refrigerated (Pillsbury):		
Apple or blueberry	1 turnover	305
Cherry	1 turnover	310
TWINKIE (Hostess):		
Regular	1 cake	149
Devil's food	1 cake	213

V

Food and Description	Measure or Quantity	Sodium (mgs.)
VEAL, broiled, medium cooked:		
Loin chop	4 oz.	91
Rib, roasted	4 oz.	91
Steak or cutlet, lean & fat	4 oz.	91
VEAL DINNER, frozen:		
(Banquet):		
Buffet Supper	2-lb. pkg.	6599
Dinner, regular	11-oz. dinner	2527
(Swanson):		
Hungry Man, parmigiana	20½-oz. dinner	2190
TV Brand, parmigiana	12¼-oz. dinner	970
(Weight Watchers) parmigiana, 2-compartment	9-oz. meal	1084
VEGETABLE BOUILLON		
(Herb-Ox):		
Cube	1 cube	920
Packet	1 packet	880
VEGETABLE JUICE COCKTAIL:		
Regular, *V-8*	6 fl. oz.	640
Dietetic:		
(S&W) *Nutradiet*, low sodium	6 fl. oz.	25
V-8, low sodium	6 fl. oz.	60
VEGETABLES, MIXED:		
Canned, regular pack:		
(Del Monte) drained	½ cup	309
(La Choy) Chinese	1 cup	99
(Libby's) solids & liq.	½ cup	345
Canned, dietetic pack (Featherweight)	½ cup	25
Frozen:		
(Birds Eye):		
Regular:		
Broccoli, cauliflower & carrots in cheese sauce	3⅓ oz.	316
Carrots, peas & onions deluxe	3⅓ oz.	53

119

Food and Description	Measure or Quantity	Sodium (mgs.)
Mixed	3⅓ oz.	38
With onion sauce	2.7 oz.	335
Pea & cauliflower with cream sauce	3⅓ oz.	377
Pea & pearl onion	3⅓ oz.	311
Pea & potato with cream sauce	2.7 oz.	490
Stew	6.7 oz.	49
Blue Ribbon:		
Broccoli, carrots & potato in lightly seasoned sauce	3⅓ oz.	262
Corn, green beans & pasta in lightly seasoned sauce	3⅓ oz.	282
Mixed	3⅓ oz.	278
Farm Fresh:		
Broccoli, cauliflower & carrot strips	3.2 oz.	21
Brussels sprouts, cauliflower & carrots	3.2 oz.	17
International Style:		
Chinese style	⅓ of pkg.	360
Italian style	⅓ of pkg.	574
Japanese style	⅓ of pkg.	502
Mexican style	⅓ of pkg.	462
Stir Fry:		
Cantonese style	⅓ of pkg.	469
Chinese style	⅓ of pkg.	497
Japanese style	⅓ of pkg.	530
(Green Giant):		
Regular:		
Broccoli, cauliflower & carrots in cheese sauce	3⅓ oz.	390
Mixed	3⅓ oz.	44
Mixed, in butter sauce	3⅓ oz.	287
Pea, pod & water chestnuts in butter sauce	3 oz.	308
Harvest Fresh	4 oz.	222
Harvest Get Togethers:		
Broccoli-cauliflower medley	3⅓ oz.	388
Cauliflower-carrot bonanza	3⅓ oz.	245
Chinese style	3⅓ oz.	234
Japanese style	3⅓ oz.	118
(La Choy):		
Chinese	5-oz. serving	777
Japanese	5-oz. serving	612

Food and Description	Measure or Quantity	Sodium (mgs.)
(Le Seuer) pea, carrot & onion in butter sauce	3⅓ oz.	85
VEGETABLES IN PASTRY, frozen (Pepperidge Farm):		
Asparagus with mornay sauce	3¾ oz.	245
Broccoli with cheese	3¾ oz.	455
Cauliflower with cheese sauce	3¾ oz.	465
Spinach almondine	3¾ oz.	325
Zucchini provencal	3¾ oz.	290
VEGETABLE STEW, canned, *Dinty Moore*	7½-oz. serving	967
"VEGETARIAN FOODS":		
Canned or dry:		
Chicken, fried (Loma Linda) with gravy	1½-oz. piece	217
Chili (Worthington)	¼ can (5-oz. serving)	695
Choplet (Worthington)	1 choplet	263
Dinner cuts (Loma Linda) drained	1 cut	273
Franks, big (Loma Linda)	1.9-oz. frank	437
Franks, sizzle (Loma Linda)	2.2-oz. frank	406
FriChik (Worthington)	1 piece	277
Granburger (Worthington)	6 T.	998
Little links (Loma Linda) drained	.8-oz. link	139
Non-meatballs (Worthington)	1 meatball	342
Proteena (Loma Linda)	½" slice	523
Sandwich spread:		
(Loma Linda)	1 T.	134
Concentrate, liquid	1 cup	178
Ready to use	1 cup	84
Soyameat (Worthington):		
Sliced beef	1 slice	140
Salisbury steak	1 slice	403
Stew pack (Loma Linda) drained	1 piece	44
Super links (Worthington)	1 link	559
Swiss steak with gravy (Loma Linda)	1 steak	482
Tender bits (Loma Linda) drained	1 piece	163
Vegelona (Loma Linda)	½" slice	494
Vega-Links (Worthington)	1 link	206
Worthington 209	1 slice	229
Frozen:		
Beef-like slices (Worthington)	1 slice	140
Beef pie (Worthington)	1 pie	15,679
Bologna (Loma Linda)	1 oz.	304
Chicken (Loma Linda)	1 slice	281

Food and Description	Measure or Quantity	Sodium (mgs.)
Chicken, fried (Loma Linda)	2-oz. serving	289
Chicken pie (Worthington)	1 pie	15,811
FriPats (Worthington)	1 pat	607
Meatballs (Loma Linda)	1 meatball	253
Prosage (Worthington)	1 link	227
Roast Beef (Loma Linda)	1 oz.	319
Sausage, breakfast (Loma Linda)	⅓" slice	250
Turkey (Loma Linda)	1 oz.	281
VERMOUTH (Great Western) dry & sweet	1 fl. oz.	7
VICHY WATER (Schweppa)	6 fl. oz.	80
VIENNA SAUSAGE:		
(Hormel):		
Regular	1 sausage	155
Chicken	1-oz. serving	237
(Libby's) in beef broth	1 link (.6 oz.)	94
VINEGAR	1 T.	1

W

Food and Description	Measure or Quantity	Sodium (mgs.)
WAFFELOS, cereal (Ralston Purina)	1 cup	118
WAFFLE, frozen:		
(Aunt Jemima) jumbo	1 waffle	261
(Eggo):		
Regular or strawberry	1 waffle	265
Blueberry	1 waffle	260
(Roman Meal)	1 waffle	325
WALNUT, English or Persian (Diamond A)	1 cup	2
WATER CHESTNUT, canned (La Choy) drained	¼ of 8-oz. can	Tr.
WATERCRESS, trimmed	½ cup	8
WATERMELON:		
Wedge	4" × 8" wedge	4
Diced	½ cup	1
WELSH RAREBIT:		
Home recipe	1 cup	770
Frozen (Stouffer's)	5-oz. serving	660
WESTERN DINNER, frozen:		
(Banquet)	11-oz. dinner	2178

Food and Description	Measure or Quantity	Sodium (mgs.)
(Morton) *Round-Up*	11.8-oz. dinner	1679
(Swanson):		
Hungry Man	17¾-oz. dinner	2010
TV Brand	11¾-oz. dinner	1215
WHEATENA, cereal	¼ cup	5
WHEAT FLAKES CEREAL		
(Featherweight)	1¼ cups	5
WHEAT GERM, raw (Elam's)	1 oz.	5
WHEAT GERM CEREAL		
(Kretschmer):		
Regular	¼ cup	1
Brown sugar & honey	¼ cup	3
***WHEAT HEARTS,** cereal (General		
Mills)	¾ cup	410
WHEATIES, cereal	1 cup	370
WHEAT & OATMEAL, cereal, hot		
(Elam's)	1 oz.	11
WILD BERRY DRINK, canned		
(Hi-C)	6 fl. oz.	5
WINE, COOKING (Regina):		
Burgundy or sauterne	¼ cup	365
Sherry	¼ cup	370

Y

Food and Description	Measure or Quantity	Sodium (mgs.)
YEAST, BAKER'S (Fleischmann's):		
Dry, active	¼ oz.	7
Fresh & household, active	.6-oz. cake	5
YOGURT:		
Regular:		
Plain:		
(Dannon)	8-oz. container	115
Yoplait	6-oz. container	135
Plain with honey, *Yoplait, Custard*		
Style	6-oz. container	110
Apple:		
(Dannon) Dutch	8-oz. container	70-125
Mélangé (Dannon)	6-oz. container	120
Yoplait (General Mills)	6-oz. container	120

Food and Description	Measure or Quantity	Sodium (mgs.)
Banana:		
(Dannon)	8-oz. container	70-125
Berry, *Yoplait*:		
Regular	6-oz. container	95
Mixed	6-oz. container	120
Blueberry:		
(Dannon)	8-oz. container	70-125
Mélangé	6-oz. container	120
(Sweet'n Low)	8-oz. container	170
Yoplait (General Mills)	6-oz. container	120
Yoplait, Custard style	6-oz. container	105
Boysenberry:		
(Dannon)	8-oz. container	70-125
(Sweet'N Low)	8-oz. container	170
Cherry:		
(Dannon)	8-oz. container	70-125
Mélangé	6-oz. container	120
(Sweet'N Low)	8-oz. container	170
Yoplait	6-oz. container	120
Citrus, *Yoplait, Breakfast Yogurt*	6-oz. container	95
Coffee (Dannon)	8-oz. container	70-90
Lemon:		
(Dannon)	8-oz. container	70-90
(Sweet'N Low)	8-oz. container	170
Yoplait:		
Regular	6-oz. container	120
Custard style	6-oz. container	105
Orange, *Yoplait*	6-oz. container	120
Orchard, *Yoplait, Breakfast Yogurt*	6-oz. container	95
Peach:		
(Dannon)	8-oz. container	70-125
Yoplait	6-oz. container	170
Peach melba (Colombo)	8-oz. container	120
Piña Colada:		
(Dannon)	8-oz. container	70-125
Yoplait	6-oz. container	120
Pineapple *Mélangé*	6-oz. container	120
Raspberry:		
(Dannon) red	8-oz. container	70-125
(Friendship)	8-oz. container	70-125
Mélangé	6-oz. container	120
(Sweet'N Low)	8-oz. container	120
Yoplait	6-oz. container	120
Yoplait, Custard style	6-oz. container	105

![SIGNET logo]

Staying Healthy with SIGNET Books

Buy them at your local

bookstore or use coupon

on next page for ordering.

Medical Reference Books from SIGNET

SIGNET Books for Your Reference Shelf

Recommended Reading from SIGNET

Food and Description	Measure or Quantity	Sodium (mgs.)
Strawberry:		
(Dannon)	8-oz. container	70-125
Mélangé	6-oz. container	120
(Sweet'N Low)	8-oz. container	170
Yoplait	6-oz. container	120
Strawberry banana (Sweet'N Low)	8-oz. container	170
Tropical fruit (Sweet'N Low)	8-oz. container	170
Vanilla:		
(Dannon)	8-oz. container	70-90
Yoplait, Custard style	6-oz. container	110
Frozen, hard:		
Boysenberry *Danny-On-A-Stick*, carob coated	2½-fl.-oz. bar	15
Boysenberry swirl (Bison)		
Cherry vanilla (Bison)		
Chocolate *Danny-On-A-Stick*, chocolate coated	2½-fl.-oz. bar	15
Raspberry, red (Dannon) *Danny-On-A-Stick*, chocolate coated	2½-fl.-oz. bar	15

Z

ZITI, frozen (Weight Watchers)	12½-oz. pkg.	1261
ZWIEBACK (Gerber)	1 piece	16

SIGNET Books of Special Interest

Buy them at your local

bookstore or use coupon

on next page for ordering.